Revised Edition

Truck Drivers:
Stop Your Job from Killing You!

The Dietitians' Guide to Smart Eating
and Healthy Living for Truckers

By Sharon Madalis, MS, RDN, LDN, CDE
and April Rudat, MS Ed, RDN, LDN

Published by

April Rudat, Registered Dietitian LLC

Moscow, Pennsylvania

First published 2010
Copyright © 2010, 2019 by Sharon Madalis and April Rudat

Published by
April Rudat, Registered Dietitian LLC
Moscow, Pennsylvania
www.DietitianApril.com

Library of Congress Cataloging-in-Publication Data
Control Number: 2019910211
Madalis, Sharon, & Rudat, April.
    Truck Drivers: Stop Your Job from Killing You! The Dietitians' Guide to Smart Eating and Healthy Living for Truckers / Sharon Madalis & April Rudat. -Revised ed.
    Includes references and index.
    ISBN–13: 978-0-9791549-2-8
    ISBN–10: 0-9791549-2-8

Author headshots/interior photos by Bob Calin
Book cover design/cover photo by Kristen Conniff
Revised book cover design by Stephanie Jordan,
rockpaperdesigns@gmail.com

Printed in the United States of America

For truck drivers, as you begin your road to good health.

To my husband, Ed, for his love and support. To my mom, Carol, for giving me a passion for reading and writing. To April, for helping make a dream come true.

– Sharon Madalis

To my husband, Todd, and our children, Julia and David. Thank you for your patience and love during this journey. And to Sharon, thank you for this opportunity and for your mentorship and friendship through the years.

– April Rudat

Acknowledgements

Many thanks to our trucker friends, especially Michael Travis, who not only served as our truck driver model on the cover and within the book, but also read the book, provided input, and followed the book's recommendations, which led to a 20 lb. weight loss.

Thanks also to Kristin Meredick Travis, wife of trucker Michael Travis and sister of co-author April Rudat, for ensuring that our trucker model Mike was well dressed and picture-perfect.

Thanks to Kevin Rudat, for his careful review of our manuscript and valuable input on our first draft.

Thanks to our editor, Leslie Westman, for her invaluable improvements and for helping us to say things the way we meant to say them.

Thanks to our artist, Kristen Conniff, for the adventure that led to our beautiful cover and front cover photograph, for your artistic talent, and for your cover input.

Thanks to Bob Calin for our photographs inside the book (which included a wild goose chase to get that rig in the photo!).

Thanks to our artist, Stephanie Jordan, for the book cover design updates for our revised edition.

Contents

Introduction

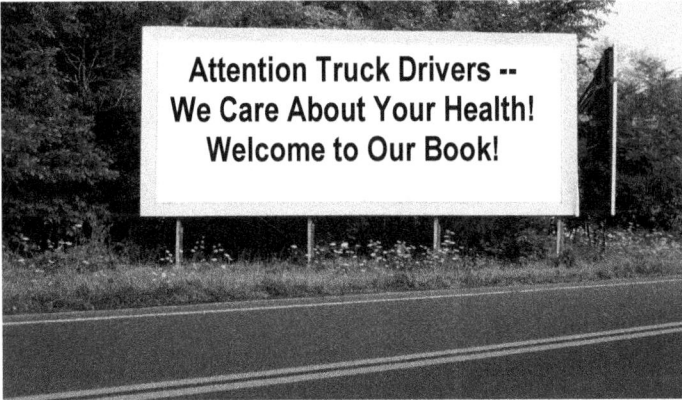

**Attention Truck Drivers --
We Care About Your Health!
Welcome to Our Book!**

This is the first in a series of books addressing how some occupations can be hazardous to your physical health. Whether your job has caused you health problems or places you at risk for health problems, this book has answers for you.

The key question is <u>how</u> can you improve your health through good nutrition and physical activity, manage or prevent diseases and conditions, and, most importantly, remain productive <u>and</u> feel good doing your job?

As health care professionals, it is easy for us to tell our clients <u>what</u> to do to improve their health based on all the scientific knowledge we gain during our training and education. As registered dietitian nutritionists, we use the skills to show clients "how to" do it. But we can do this even better when we learn more about individual lifestyles, including work habits.

One of my realizations about the importance of understanding clients' work habits came early in my career when I was counseling a big, burly truck driver who had had a heart attack. I was educating him on a heart healthy diet and stressing the need for him to eat at "better" restaurants when on the road. In other words, I was encouraging him to stop at restaurants that would offer more variety and perhaps, lower fat food choices on the menu. Without missing a beat, he growled, "Lady, where am I supposed to park my rig?" I humbled myself by recognizing that it had not occurred to me that "better" restaurants did not usually have parking lots big enough for 18-wheelers.

That truck driver did not know how his words opened my eyes to help me realize that it is not always easy to change our lifestyle habits, especially when our jobs have obstacles that may get in the way. [Sharon Madalis]

Importance of Truck Drivers

According to the U.S. Bureau of Labor Statistics, there were about 3.2 million commercial truck drivers nationwide in 2016. This includes big rig operators hauling heavy goods long distances and light or delivery services truck drivers transporting merchandise within a specific area (1).

Job growth is expected to be steady with a projected employment of 3.4 million commercial truck drivers by 2026 (1). Truck drivers will be a constant presence on our highways. After all, who else can we rely on to pick up and deliver goods door-to-door in the shortest amount of time? But what about the special health challenges truckers face?

Health Problems in Truckers

The working conditions of truck drivers put them at risk for poor health. These conditions include: long hours, stressful road conditions, periods of inactivity followed by physical demands such as heavy lifting, lack of a regular meal schedule and access to healthy foods, and poor food choices used to fight fatigue and boredom.

Studies show that about 69 percent of long-haul truck drivers are obese (2). This puts them at risk for diseases associated with excess weight, which include heart disease, high blood pressure, strokes, type 2 diabetes, and sleep disorders such as sleep apnea. Sedentary lifestyles, especially in long-haul drivers, and limited access to disease-fighting foods such as fruits and vegetables can worsen these health risks (3).

Women truck drivers are not immune to these health problems. Additional health problems reported by women truckers include sinus problems, back pain, and migraine headaches (4).

How This Book Can Help You

This book is a guide to help you educate yourself on better eating and exercise habits, which will help protect your health as you do your important job. Each chapter will give you strategies to help you make simple but important changes.

In chapter 1, you will learn what it is about your job that makes it so hazardous to your health. To help you start tackling these hazards, chapter 2 will show you what you should include in your diet every day. A common problem on the road is having to rely on meals and snacks away from home. So, chapters 3 and 4 will provide you with healthier choices when eating at restaurants and for packing your rig.

Your lifestyle as a trucker may put you at risk for being overweight and for developing health problems such as heart disease and diabetes. In chapter 5, you will learn how to manage your weight. Chapter 6 will address ways to lower cholesterol levels and blood pressure to prevent or treat heart disease; chapter 7 will help you manage your blood sugars to prevent or treat diabetes.

To help you fight fatigue while driving long hours, chapter 8 will provide healthy strategies for staying energized. Chapter 9 will continue with one major strategy, physical activity, for staying alert and improving your health. And in the final chapter, you will learn how to make other lifestyle changes, such as healthy eating while quitting tobacco or while stressed.

So that you can continue educating yourself on these important topics, we have included some useful websites and resources in the back of the book.

We Depend on You! We Care about You!

We hope that you are able to use the strategies in this book on your road to good health. After all, our country depends on you to stay in shape. Think about it: Where would America be without truck drivers?

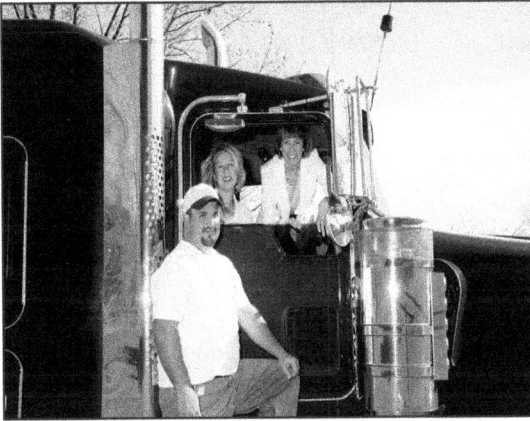

(Authors April Rudat and Sharon Madalis in the rig,
with truck driver Michael Travis.)

References

1. U.S. Bureau of Labor Statistics, Occupational Outlook Handbook. Truck drivers and drivers/sales workers. Heavy and tractor-trailer truck drivers. Available at: https://www.bls.gov-ooh/. Accessed September 9, 2018.

2. Sieber WK, et al. Obesity and other risk factors: The National Survey of U. S. long haul truck driver's health and injury. *Am J Ind Med.* 2014;57(6): 615-626.

3. Whitfield Jacobson PJ, Prawitz AD, Lukaszuk JM. Long-haul truck drivers want healthful meal options at truck-stop restaurants. *J Am Diet Assoc.* 2007;107(12):2125-2129.

4. Reed DB, Cronin JS. Health on the road: Issues faced by female truck drivers. *AAOHN J.* 2003;51(3):120-125.

Chapter 1:

Why is it So Hard for a Truck Driver to Stay Healthy?

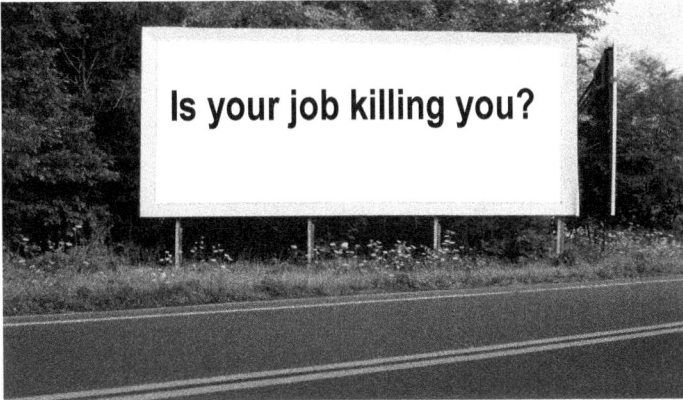

Driving trucks: It is a free-spirited and amazing career. With your window rolled down, you can experience the beauty of every region of the country. You have the opportunity to meet new and interesting people, and you get to work in the outdoors. But when you are on the road, you probably notice a number of health challenges. Let's examine some of the reasons why it is so hard for a truck driver to stay healthy.

Your Driving Environment

Riding in your cab means a lot of sitting, eating your meals on the go, and not being able to exercise or move your body very much between stops. Over time, the combination of these factors may negatively impact your weight and health.

Not Enough Exercise

Time constraints due to tight delivery schedules can leave little time for exercise. But you may be thinking, "I exercise when I'm unloading the truck." While lifting and moving heavy boxes or items for a 20-minute time span does burn some energy, this type of movement is more like strength training rather than cardiovascular exercise. Strength training is beneficial, but it is also important to exercise your heart with cardiovascular exercise such as walking, biking, or swimming. In addition, if you do have the time and want to walk at a rest stop or do laps around your truck, you may have safety concerns in certain areas, which may prevent exercise.

Poor Food Choices

Whether dining in a restaurant or carrying a brown bag, you may be making poor food choices without even realizing it. Perhaps you have never learned nutrition basics or don't believe that healthy food *can* taste good. You may not make the best food choices out of habit. Added to that is the challenge of finding healthy food while on the road.

Fast Food

Do you choose a lot of fast food out of convenience? Do you drive for a food company and then receive free food as a perk?

These circumstances can lead to weight gain and other health problems if you are not making nutrition-conscious choices.

Restaurants

Perhaps you stop at truck stops for a nice, home-cooked meal. Hot-cooked meals at truck stop restaurants seem healthy, right? Not always. These meals may be smothered in butter and gravies. The cuts of meat may be fatty, and the side dishes and large desserts can lead to overeating and possible weight gain.

One reason why eating out can be hazardous to your health is that the meals can contain hidden fats and salt. Plain and simple, the hot-cooked meals at truck stop restaurants may be no healthier than meals at fast food restaurants.

No Parking Spot for Your Truck

So why not dine at a health-conscious café? While following this suggestion can improve your nutritional choices, it is often not realistic. There may be no parking spot for your rig, the service is likely not fast enough for your busy schedule, and the price may not be as appealing as the food.

Frequent Snacking

Another road hazard to your health is frequent snacking in your rig. You may snack throughout your entire shift out of boredom or just to stay awake. If you are munching on salty snacks or sugar-laden sweets and eating when you do not have actual hunger, you may be overeating without even realizing it. This can eventually lead to unwanted weight gain.

Lack of Fruits, Vegetables, and Whole Grains

A diet rich in fruits, vegetables, and whole grains can provide many health benefits such as decreasing your risk of certain cancers and helping to manage your weight. However, you may not think to include many of these foods in your diet. Or, you may have trouble finding them on the road or fitting them into your food budget (1). Without them in your diet, you miss the potential health benefits they offer.

Risky Beverage Choices

What is your beverage choice? Soda, sports or energy drinks, coffee? Drinking large amounts of any sweetened beverages like soda, sweetened tea, lemonade, fruit punch and naturally sweetened drinks like juice can pack on the pounds. Think about it this way: Would you rather eat your calories or drink them? Most people would rather eat the food.

Science has taught us that the liquid calories in sweetened beverages do not give us the same fullness as when we chew our food. Therefore, consuming drinks with calories daily can lead to weight gain.

Timing of Meals

If your shift starts at 1:00 am, when are you supposed to eat "breakfast?" Eating at irregular times and skipping meals are common habits of shift workers that can negatively influence health (2). In addition, working at times when your body and mind are set to sleep can be tough on your body, leading to chronic sleep problems, weight changes, stomach problems, and even heart disease (2).

Long Hours/Shift Work

As you know, long hours or working through the night can make your job downright tiring. You may have needed to adjust your sleep schedule based on the shifts you work, or you may get less sleep than you need overall. Being chronically sleep deprived makes some of our body's hormones trigger us to overeat. The fact is: Regular sleep is an important part of health, especially for someone who works as hard as you do in the trucking industry.

Stress

If you are under time constraints for making deliveries, you may feel high levels of stress. You may be forced to choose fast foods, and you may need to eat your food quickly. Sometimes you may eat emotionally just to relieve stress. All of these factors can negatively affect your health.

Lack of Health Insurance

With the rising cost of fuel, truckers may face another challenge: less money for health insurance coverage or no health insurance at all. Not having health insurance makes it very difficult to keep up with important health screenings and pay for necessary medical procedures.

Bad Habits

Do you smoke? Do you use chewing tobacco or a pipe? Do you use supplements or herbals to stay awake? Do you sometimes dabble in drugs? Do you have excessive stress or anger? All of these can impact your health in serious ways.

Our Mission

Where would we be without truck drivers? We, the authors, value your work, and we also value your health. Therefore, throughout this book, we hope you will learn simple eating and exercise tips to improve your health and quality of life.

Worksite Wellness

We must also mention one important piece of advice: If your employer has a worksite wellness program, take advantage of it. Have your blood pressure, cholesterol, blood sugar, and weight checked if such screenings are offered. Take advantage of tobacco cessation, healthy eating, and healthy lifestyle presentations if they are offered. Also, if you have a chance to meet with Registered Dietitian Nutritionists (RDNs), Registered Nurses (RNs), or the Wellness Coaches within your company, do so.

References

1. Lincoln JE et al. A pilot study of healthy living options at 16 truck stops across the United States. *Am J Health Promot.* 2018; 32(3):546-553.
2. Sawyer-Morse MK. Lunch at midnight: The impact of shift work on health. *Today's Dietitian.* 2006; 8(6):55-56.

Chapter 2:
Trucker Nutrition Basics

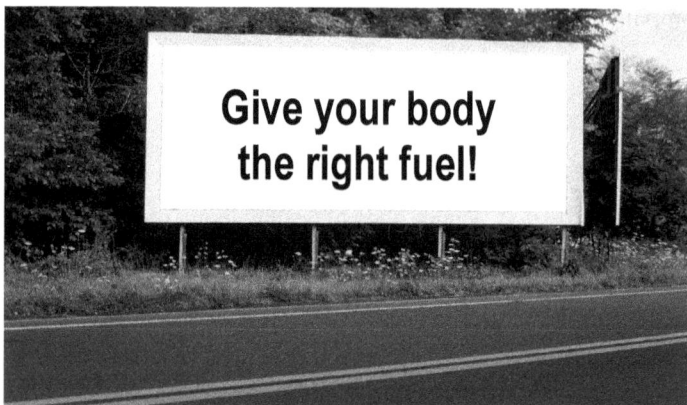

Give your body
the right fuel!

Any smart trucker knows that fueling your rig <u>and</u> doing routine maintenance and repairs on your rig are important if you want your truck to keep running smoothly. What is true for your truck is also true for your body. If you don't give yourself the right fuel (food) and maintain and repair your body, you will eventually have trouble keeping up with your schedule and run into health problems down the road.

ChooseMyPlate:
Fuel for your body
A good place to start to see if you are using the right fuel is to compare your current diet to the MyPlate.

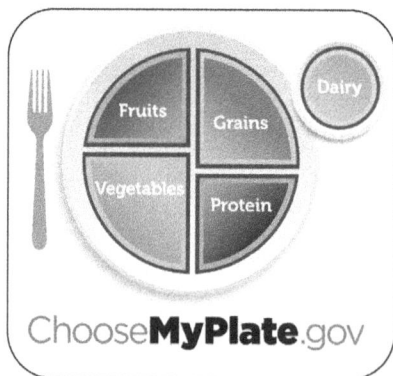

(Source: U. S. Department of Agriculture)

MyPlate is a simple tool that gives you the basic foods and amounts necessary for your daily diet. You can get personalized information by visiting ChooseMyPlate.gov.

With the chart we have provided below, you can also keep a food log for one day, recording all food and beverages and the exact amounts you ate and drank. Next, compare what you ate to the recommended servings per day from MyPlate.

My Food Log	Recommended Servings
Time Food /Drink Amount	**Check a box for each serving you had:** **Fruit** ☐ ☐ (1 serving: 1 piece or 1 cup fruit) **Vegetables** ☐ ☐ ☐ (1 serving: 1 cup raw or cooked) **Grains** ☐ ☐ ☐ ☐ ☐ ☐ (1 serving: 1 ounce; at least 3 ounces as whole grain choices) **Dairy** ☐ ☐ ☐ (1 serving: 1 cup) **Protein (Meat)** ☐ ☐ ☐ ☐ ☐ ☐ (6 ounces/day) **Fats and Oils** ☐ ☐ ☐ ☐ ☐ ☐ (6 teaspoons/day) **Water** ☐ ☐ ☐ ☐ (At least four, 16-ounce glasses a day) **Exercise** ☐ (30-60 minutes/day)

What Should I Eat? What's a Serving?

If you are like most people, you may not know serving sizes. You also may not always know which foods belong to which group or how much of each group you should be eating every day. Let's take a closer look at the nutrients you need to maintain a healthy body, the foods that provide those nutrients, what we mean by a "serving," and how many servings you should strive for daily.

Carbohydrates

Carbohydrates provide the best source of energy to fuel your body and are the main fuel source for your brain. In fact, half of the calories you eat should come from carbohydrate foods. Here are the other important roles of carbohydrates:

- regulate your blood sugar
- provide fiber that can protect against certain cancers and heart disease
- help you feel full
- relieve constipation

Carbohydrates are found in fruit, vegetables, grains, milk and yogurt. These are carbohydrates that carry you for the "long haul." Sugars and sweets also contain carbohydrates, but these foods are more processed so they have less vitamins, minerals, and fiber compared to the other carbohydrate foods and would only carry you for the "short haul." Keep these foods for just once in a while.

Here are some serving sizes of carbohydrates from MyPlate:

Fruit: 1 cup fresh or canned fruit, 1 medium-sized fruit, ½ cup dried fruit (like raisins or dried apricots), 1 cup 100% fruit juice (limit juice to 1 cup per day)

Vegetables: 1 cup raw or cooked vegetables, 1 cup vegetable juice, 2 cups raw leafy greens (Note: Starchy vegetables like potatoes, corn, and lima beans contain more carbohydrate than other vegetables.)

Grains: 1 slice bread, 1 small tortilla, 1 cup ready-to-eat cereal (like shredded wheat), ½ cup cooked cereal (like oatmeal), ½ cup cooked rice or pasta, 3 cups light popped popcorn

Dairy: 1 cup (8 oz.) milk, 1 cup yogurt, 1 cup pudding

The amount you need from each of these food groups will vary depending on your age, gender, your weight goals (lose, maintain, or gain weight), and physical activity level.

Here are your daily suggested carbohydrate servings:

Fruit: 2 cups a day -- Vary your fruit choices and aim for more fresh fruit.

Vegetables: 3 cups a day -- Vary your vegetable choices and eat more dark green and orange vegetables.

Grains: 6 ounces a day -- Choose more whole grains such as whole wheat bread, oatmeal, and brown rice.

Dairy: 3 cups a day -- Choose low-fat dairy products more often.

Protein

Protein serves as building material for growth and repair of your body. Additionally, protein:

- helps your body fight infection and heal properly
- builds and maintains muscle

Protein is found in meat such as chicken, turkey, fish, beef, veal, pork, lamb and game meat. It is also in "meat substitutes" such as eggs, milk, yogurt, cheese, tofu, beans such as kidney beans or black beans, lentils, and nuts, seeds, and peanut butter.

Here are some serving sizes of protein foods:

Meat: 1-ounce meat, poultry, or fish

Meat substitutes: 1 cup milk or yogurt, 1 ½ ounce cheese (use low-fat dairy products), 2 ounces processed cheese, 1 egg, 1 Tablespoon peanut butter, 1 Tablespoon nuts or seeds, ¼ cup cooked dry beans/lentils, ¼ cup tofu, 2 Tablespoons hummus

The amount you need from each of these food groups will vary depending on your age, gender, weight goals (lose, maintain, or gain weight), and physical activity level. Some medical conditions may require more or less protein in the diet. Interestingly, the amount of carbohydrate in the diet plays a role in allowing protein to perform its tasks of building and repairing. Without adequate carbohydrate, protein will be tapped for energy, which is not its optimal job.

Here are suggested servings a day from proteins:

Meat and meat substitutes: 6 ounces a day -- Choose skinless poultry, fish, lean meats, and low-fat dairy foods. A 3-ounce piece of meat, poultry, or fish equals the size of a deck of cards.

Fat

Fat is known as the storage nutrient. Most of the fat we eat gets stored in our body to use for energy when the body has used up the fuel or calories from carbohydrate. We need to be careful not to eat too much fat, or we will store too much. Not all fats are created equal; in Chapter 6, you will learn how to choose heart healthy options for fats.

Other important roles of fat include:
- insulates your body to protect against temperature extremes
- cushions body organs
- carries important vitamins through the body
- helps you feel full

Fat is found in some protein foods and whole milk dairy products. It is basic to ingredients that give food flavor and moisture such as margarine, butter, oil, mayonnaise, salad dressing, nuts, and olives.

Here are some serving sizes of fats:

Fats, Oils, and Dressings: 1 teaspoon soft-tub margarine or butter, 1 teaspoon oil, 1 teaspoon mayonnaise, 1 Tablespoon salad dressing, 1 Tablespoon nuts, 5 olives

(Note: 1 Tablespoon = 3 teaspoons)

The number of servings you need from fats will vary depending on your age, gender, weight goals (lose, maintain, or gain weight), and physical activity level.

In general, here are suggested servings a day from fats:

Fats: 6 teaspoons a day -- Choose unsaturated fats (fats from plant sources, such as vegetable oils, olives, avocados, and nuts) and limit the amount of fats added to foods. Instead of butter or stick margarine, choose light soft-tub or squeeze margarine with no trans fat. Healthier oils include olive, canola, and peanut oils. But remember: Even healthy oils are still fats, so use in moderation only. Finally, avoid fried foods and deep-frying cooking methods.

Portion Distortion

If you are like most people, you may not be eating the actual suggested serving size from each food group. Most likely, you may be eating a "portion" size, which is usually much larger than the recommended serving size.

This may happen at a restaurant where you are served portions that are actually equal to the serving sizes for three people. If you are eating out of boredom or choosing foods that don't fill you up, especially when it comes to snacks, you may be grabbing extra large portions. This is called "portion distortion" and can lead to problems with managing your weight and other health problems over time.

To help you get a better handle on how much you are eating, start by measuring your foods using measuring cups and spoons when you are home. Or, simply use an eight-inch plate and divide it up like a MyPlate. If the serving sizes seem too small for you, at least start cutting back compared to what you normally eat. For example, take 1 to 2 Tablespoons less than what you usually take. Try doing the following:

- Use smaller plates, bowls, and drinking glasses.
- Serve from the counter or stove rather than family style.
- Avoid extreme hunger: Eat at regularly scheduled meal times, about every 4 hours. If you are expecting long delays between meals, plan to eat some healthy snacks.
- Never eat foods directly out of the original containers. Always use small cups or dishes to serve food.

Determining Portion Sizes

When you are traveling, it may be hard for you to measure your food. But you can eyeball food to estimate how much you are eating and compare your portion size to objects that are familiar to you. The "hand" images on the next page can help you determine approximate serving sizes

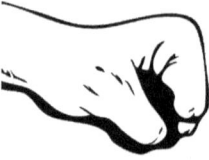

Small Fist = 1 cup

If you have a large hand, your fist may actually = 2 cups.

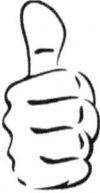

Small Thumb = 1 Tablespoon

If you have a large hand, your thumb may actually = 2 Tablespoons.

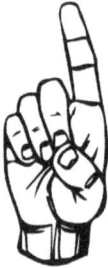

Small Fingertip = 1 teaspoon

If you have a large hand, your fingertip may actually = 2 teaspoons.

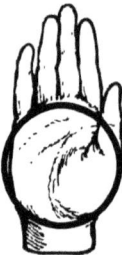

Small Palm of Hand = 3 ounces (for meat portions)

If you have a large hand, your palm may actually = 6 ounces.

Food Labels

The Nutrition Facts label on all packaged food can also help you learn more appropriate serving sizes. Here is a sample label and some simple rules to follow.

Nutrition Facts

8 servings per container
Serving size   2/3 cup (55g)

Pay attention to the Serving size.

Amount per serving
Calories   230

	% Daily Value*
Total Fat 8g	**10%**
Saturated Fat 1g	**5%**
Trans Fat 0g	
Cholesterol 0mg	**0%**
Sodium 160mg	**7%**
Total Carbohydrate 37g	**13%**
Dietary Fiber 4g	**14%**
Total Sugars 12g	
Includes 10g Added Sugars	**20%**
Protein 3g	
Vitamin D 2mcg	10%
Calcium 260mg	20%
Iron 8mg	45%
Potassium 240mg	6%

* The % Daily Value (DV) tells you how much a nutrient in a serving of food contributes to a daily diet. 2,000 calories a day is used for general nutrition advice.

Source: FDA.gov, FOR REFERENCE ONLY

Choose foods with less than 5% of the Daily Value for Saturated Fat, Trans Fat, and Cholesterol.

Choose foods with under 140 mg Sodium or less than 5% of the Daily Value.

Choose foods with more than 10% of the Daily Value for dietary fiber, vitamins, and minerals.

Limit added sugars to less than 10% of total calories daily.

Putting It All Together

If you are really struggling with knowing what to eat, here are two sample menus to follow to help you get started:

Menu #1:	Menu #2:
Breakfast 1 cup cooked oatmeal 2 Tablespoons nuts or seeds ½ cup of berries 1 cup low-fat milk	**Breakfast** Small whole grain bagel 2 teaspoons soft-tub margarine 2 eggs 1 small banana
Lunch 2 slices rye bread 3 slices (3 ounces) turkey 2 teaspoons mayonnaise 1 cup raw vegetables such as carrots 1 cup low-fat yogurt Medium-size pear	**Lunch** 1 whole grain bun ½ cup tuna 2 teaspoons mayonnaise 1 cup vegetable soup 1 cup low-fat milk
	Afternoon Snack 1 mozzarella cheese stick 6 whole wheat crackers
Dinner 3 ounces lean beef (size of a deck of cards) 1 cup brown rice 1 cup steamed green beans 1 teaspoon soft-tub margarine 1 cup tossed salad 2 Tablespoons salad dressing 1 cup low-fat milk	**Dinner** 3 ounces broiled salmon (size of a deck of cards) Small baked potato 1 cup steamed peas 2 teaspoons soft-tub margarine 1 cup pudding
Evening Snack 3 cups light microwave popcorn Medium-size apple	**Evening Snack** 1-ounce pretzels 1 cup grapes

You can also find a grocery list in Appendix E (page 131) that you may reproduce with our permission. This will come in handy whether you or family members are shopping for groceries for meals at home or food for your rig when you are on the road.

Chapter 3:

Revamping Restaurant and Takeout Choices

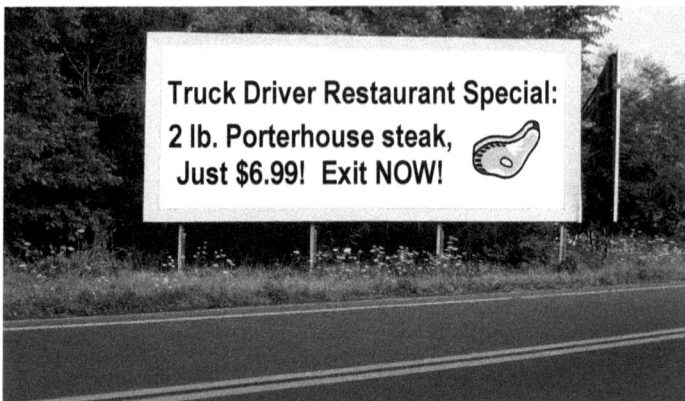

Truck Driver Restaurant Special:
2 lb. Porterhouse steak,
Just $6.99! Exit NOW!

This tantalizing message is too good to pass up, right? Wrong!
Even though a two-pound steak for $6.99 sounds like a
bargain, when it comes to health, this is a bad deal. This meal
could potentially contain more than a day's worth of heart-
clogging fat. Taking advantage of "deals" like these may lead
to serious health problems. It's just not worth it.

Think about some other common meals at truck stop
restaurants: A heaping pile of meatloaf, mashed potatoes, and
buttered corn. Greasy fried chicken, greens, and a baked potato
loaded with sour cream and butter. Mile-long buffets and
more…the list of typical truck stop restaurant food can go on
and on. But the reality is: Typical truck stop restaurant fare can

wreak havoc on your health. While some of those menu options appear harmless, they may be loaded with hidden fat and salt that can eventually affect your weight and your heart.

A research study found that many drivers would choose more nutritious options if the restaurants offered them (1). What are more nutritious options at truck stop restaurants? See our sample truck stop menu for some ideas.

Our sample truck stop menu on the next page includes typical truck stop fare. The items that we have CROSSED OUT are less healthy items – foods high in fat and sodium. All other items that are NOT CROSSED OUT are better choices on the menu. Remember to put together a MyPlate with half your plate full of fruits and vegetables. Bon Appétit!

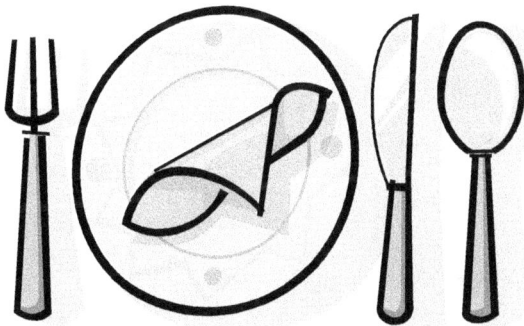

SAMPLE TRUCK STOP RESTAURANT MENU

Soups and Such!
Soup and Salad Bar $6.99
Soup and Vegetable Platter $4.99
Bowl of Chili $3.99
Chicken Noodle Soup – Cup $2.99,
Bowl $3.99
~~New England Clam Chowder – Cup~~
~~$3.99, Bowl $4.99~~
Manhattan Clam Chowder – Cup
$3.99, Bowl $4.99
Large House Salad $3.99
with Grilled Chicken $6.99
~~with Fried Chicken $6.99~~
~~with Buffalo Fried Chicken $7.99~~

* Choice of Dressings: Italian, Oil and
Vinegar, ~~Ranch,~~ ~~French,~~ Light
Ranch, Light French, Balsamic
Vinaigrette, ~~Creamy Peppercorn~~

Side Dishes/Appetizers
~~French Fries $1.99~~
Baked Potato $1.99
~~with bacon, cheese, sour~~
~~cream, and chives $3.99~~
Mashed Potatoes $1.99
~~with gravy $2.50~~
~~Hash Browns $1.99~~
~~Onion Rings $1.99~~
~~Blooming Onion $4.99~~
Steamed Vegetables $0.99
Sliced Tomatoes $0.99
Coleslaw $0.99
Cottage Cheese $1.99
~~Hot Wings $4.99~~
~~Boneless Buffalo Wings, fried $4.99~~
Shrimp Cocktail $4.99
Two Crab Cakes, broiled $5.99

Burgers
~~Double Cheeseburger with Bacon~~
~~$6.99~~
Burger with Lettuce, Tomato, Onion
$6.99
~~Burger with Double Cheese/Sauce~~
~~$6.99~~

More Burgers...
Your Choice of Chicken or Turkey
Burger, grilled & served with lettuce
& tomato $6.99
Veggie Burger $6.99

* All burgers served with choice of
one side: ~~fries, potato chips,~~
pinto beans, broth soup, or coleslaw

Entrees
Grilled Flounder, served with rice and
vegetable of the day $7.99
~~Fried Seafood Platter $7.99~~
~~Fried Catfish, with fries and coleslaw~~
~~$7.99~~
Shrimp Platter, with rice & coleslaw
Grilled $8.99, ~~Fried $7.99~~
Salmon, served with rice and
coleslaw $8.99
6 oz. Sirloin Steak, served with
choice of potato and vegetable
$7.99
~~12 oz. T-Bone Steak,~~ served with
choice of potato and vegetable
$10.99
~~Chicken Fried Steak,~~ served with
choice of potato and vegetable
$7.99
Grilled Chicken, served with choice
of potato and vegetable $7.99
~~Fried Chicken,~~ served with choice of
potato and vegetable $7.99

Desserts
One scoop ice cream $1.99
~~"Pig's Dinner:" Five scoops ice cream~~
~~$3.99~~
~~Hot Fudge Sundae $2.99~~
~~with brownie $4.99~~
~~Banana Split $2.99~~
~~Milk Shake $1.99~~
Slice of apple, pumpkin, strawberry,
~~lemon meringue, or coconut custard~~
pie $1.99
Strawberry shortcake $1.99

10 Tips for Eating Healthier at Truck Stops and Other Restaurants

1. Don't get to the restaurant too hungry so you don't overeat or overindulge: Eat snacks in between meals to avoid feeling famished.

2. Don't be afraid to request healthier options or modifications: You can ask for an item to be grilled instead of fried, you can ask for an item without butter, and you can ask that all sauces, gravies, and dressings be served on the side.

3. If you are not sure how the item is prepared, ask plenty of questions to determine if the food is healthy or not.

4. Look for heart healthy terms such as: *steamed, grilled, broiled, baked, roasted, poached,* and *lightly sautéed.*

5. Avoid foods that say: *crispy, fried, creamy, cheesy, butter sauce, hollandaise, batter dipped,* and *quick-fried.*

6. Share meals with a friend or family member, or partly fill a take-home box at the <u>beginning</u> of your meal to reduce the portion size as soon as you are served.

7. Start your meal with a broth-based soup or a salad with light or Italian dressing.

8. Ask for vegetables or fruit as a substitute if your meal comes with fries.

9. Order a healthful appetizer as your meal to cut down on your portion size.

10. Be creative with your restaurant choice. Did you know that many Wal-Mart® stores have Subway® restaurants inside, and many Target® stores have inexpensive and healthy sandwiches available? Take advantage of the easy parking and healthier options.

Choosing Healthier Breakfast Food

When it comes to lower fat and lower calorie options, breakfast can be one of the easier meals. Here are six breakfast ordering tips:

1. Instead of a 3-egg omelet, try it with an egg substitute (like Egg Beaters®) or ask for a 2-egg omelet with veggies.
2. Instead of bacon or sausage, order Canadian bacon or ham, if available. Or, try turkey bacon or turkey sausage.
3. Ask that your toast is **not** buttered so you can control how much you put on. Do the same when ordering pancakes, French toast, waffles, and biscuits.
4. Limit how much pancake syrup you use. Or, ask for light syrup, which has less sugar.
5. Watch your bagels: The big ones are equal to 4 pieces of bread. Add a protein like peanut butter to stay fuller longer.
6. Other healthy breakfast choices include whole grain cereals such as oatmeal, Wheaties®, Raisin Bran®, or Shredded Wheat®. Top them with fruit and low-fat milk, or add a fruit and cottage cheese plate to your whole grain cereal order.

Choosing Healthier Appetizers

Choosing healthier appetizers can be difficult, so here are four hints:

1. Choose broth-based soups instead of cream soups, and order a cup instead of a bowl.

2. Choose a salad with oil and vinegar-based dressing, and ask for your dressing on the side.

3. Choose fruit or vegetable appetizers that are not fried.

4. Limit your bread to one or two pieces, and spread on only a thin layer of soft-tub margarine or butter.

Choosing Healthier Entrees

Choosing a healthier entrée can be tricky at restaurants. Whether at a steakhouse, seafood restaurant, or truck stop, here are some tips based on the *type* of meat you might choose:

1. Red Meat Choices (Beef, Pork, Veal, and Lamb)

- If you choose steak, choose lean cuts: *round or flank steaks, filet mignon, sirloin,* or *London broil.*

- Choose *grilled* meat, steak, and pork rather than fried.

- Choose petite or children's portions for about three or four ounces of meat, and be sure to trim off the fat.

- Ask that sauces and butters be placed "on the side" since restaurants often top steak with butter.

- Remember: For the health of your heart, limit your red meat to less than twice a week.

2. Poultry Choices

- Remove the skin from poultry.
- Choose *baked, grilled,* or *broiled* rather than fried poultry.
- If your chicken is served with breading, remove the breading and skin and do not eat it.

3. Seafood Choices

- Choose grilled or steamed seafood for a healthy main course; avoid the fried types.
- Try salmon or tuna, which contain beneficial fats for your heart.

Side Dishes

Side dishes can be loaded with butter, cheese, and other hidden fats. Here are six helpful hints when ordering side dishes:

1. Order steamed vegetables with soft-tub margarine on the side. Applesauce and fruit side dishes are great options too.
2. Pasta or noodles with tomato or marinara sauce are better options than pastas that are drenched in butter, cream, Alfredo, cheese, or scampi sauces.
3. Skip the macaroni and cheese, or keep the portion small.

4. Instead of potato and macaroni salads, choose a pasta salad that comes with Italian dressing on it.

5. Ask for mashed potatoes with butter and gravy on the side.

6. A baked potato can be a great option if you use only small amounts of soft-tub margarine and sour cream. Or, top your potato with salsa, light Ranch salad dressing, or ketchup instead.

Can You Make Healthier Choices at Buffets?

You can! But there are some basic tips for eating at buffets:

1. Choose small portions. Try to fill only two plates: One for salad and one for dinner. And do not make a mountain on your plate – this is not a small portion.

2. Swap your plates. If available, use a large plate for salad, fruit, and vegetables and a small plate for your entree and healthy sides.

3. Fill up on a broth-based soup and a vegetable salad with oil and vinegar-based dressing first.

4. Make healthy choices with only one or two real indulgences. Sit down, take your time eating, and enjoy your meal. Let the sample "plates" on the next page be your guide.

BUFFET PLATES:

PLATE # 2: ENTREE

AVOID:
- Fried, creamy, or cheesy choices

CHOOSE:
- Baked, grilled, or broiled entrees & steamed vegetables
- Make a MyPlate with half your plate as veggies.

CUP OF BROTH SOUP

GLASS OF WATER

PLATE # 1: SALAD PLATE

AVOID:
- Creamy dressings
- Creamy pasta salads
- Meat, bacon, and cheese toppings
- Fried items from the salad bar

CHOOSE:
- Lots of fresh vegetables/fruits
- Many colorful vegetables in your salad
- Italian or oil and vinegar-based dressings

My Buffet Experience

We would guess that not too many dietitians choose to eat at buffets. While writing this book, however, we had the opportunity to experience a buffet firsthand, and we successfully used our buffet tips mentioned earlier. We ordered unsweetened iced tea, enjoyed a cup of homemade chicken noodle soup, and then made the trip to the buffet line for salad and an entrée. Seeing many other diners' plates stacked as high as Mount Everest with fried, greasy foods, we made our quest to consume a normal-sized, healthy meal, and in the process, we made a few discoveries:

- Many people at buffets eat *quickly* so they can taste *everything*:
    - Instead, walk around the buffet before filling your plate so you can see which "healthy but tasty" options are available.
    - Then, place normal-sized portions on your two plates -- your salad plate and your dinner plate -- and eat slowly so you can taste and enjoy each part of your meal.
- Remember: You don't have to eat something if it doesn't taste good.
    - You may have been told in your life that discarding food is wasting it; but if you are eating something you do not like or

eating it to "clean your plate," you are indeed "wasting food" -- you are "wasting food" by not eating something that is enjoyable to you.

- When we "clean our plate" even though we are no longer hunger, this leads to overeating and unwanted weight gain.

• With the serving tongs or spoons, take food from the top of the pile since the food at the bottom is likely drenched in drippings, gravies, cheese sauces, or butter.

Are There Healthier Fast Food and Takeout Options?

Yes, and most fast food restaurants have nutrition facts available in the restaurant and online so you can compare products and make a better choice. Or you can go to CalorieKing.com for nutrition facts or carbohydrate content (for those with diabetes who count carbs), and other information for your favorite fast food items. For more healthy options, also check out HealthyDiningFinder.com.

So, what are basic guidelines for creating a healthier fast food meal?

---

* Create a MyPlate.
* In an <u>entire restaurant meal</u>, aim for:
   - about 500 calories
   - less than 20 grams of fat
   - less than 800 mg sodium

Enhance Your Plate

You can improve your plate by making a MyPlate at fast food restaurants:

Instead of:	Choose:
McDonalds® Quarter Pounder with Cheese "Meal" with fries and a drink	Regular cheeseburger, small fries, a packet of apple slices and water
McDonalds® Crispy Chicken or Fish Sandwich "Meal" with fries and a drink	Grilled chicken sandwich, side salad, a fruit and yogurt parfait, and water
One Dunkin donut and a medium iced latte	Veggie egg white sandwich with a plain iced coffee with low-fat milk and 1 shot of flavor sweetener
Two Slices Pepperoni Pizza Hut® Pizza	Two slices with veggie toppings and buy fruit or dried fruit to add fiber
A KFC® Meal with one chicken drumstick, one biscuit, mashed potatoes with gravy, and a drink	Kentucky grilled chicken with green beans, cole slaw, and a biscuit with a water
Wendy's® Bacon Cheeseburger with fries and a drink	Wendy's® chili with a garden side salad and a water
Taco Bell® 3 Crunchy Tacos Supreme® and pink lemonade	Two Taco Bell® Supreme soft tacos, a side of black beans, and water

(Sources: Mcdonalds.com; Dunkindonuts.com; Pizzahut.com; KFC.com; Wendys.com; Tacobell.com; respectively.)

To cut down on fast food calories, stick with grilled options and avoid fried items. Also order items plain – without the cheese, sauces, and bacon. Instead of French fries, order healthier sides like salad with oil and vinegar-based dressing or fruit options like apple slices or fruit salad. Quench your thirst with a bottle of water or another calorie-free beverage like unsweetened tea or diet drinks. And remember: order the normal portion size instead of "sizing up." "Super-sized" meals mean "super-sized" calories – that's no deal!

So, What Should You Choose?

There are healthier choices available at restaurants, so use the chart on the following page for some great tips based on different types of cuisine.

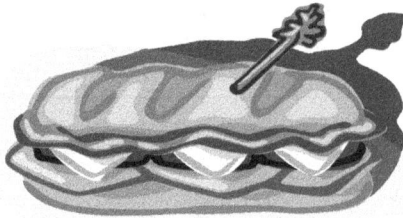

Food Type	Fast Food Restaurants	Chinese Food	Italian Food	Mexican Food
Choose	- Sub sandwiches - Grilled chicken sandwiches - Plain hamburger - Chili - Sauces like BBQ, ketchup, and honey mustard - Salads with grilled chicken - Fruit platters and yogurt parfaits - Bottled water	- Wonton, egg drop, or hot and sour soup - Broiled, steamed, or lightly stir-fried items - Items from the "Dieters" menu - Steamed rice - Steamed veggies - Non-fried sushi	- Broth soups - Salad with dressing on side - Only one or two pieces of bread - Pastas with tomato or white wine sauces - Baked fish/meats - Thin crust pizzas with veggies	- Baked or grilled items - Ask how it is prepared if you are not sure. - Salsa - Guacamole is OK, but go easy. - Traditional rice and beans - Soft tacos or fajitas instead of hard tacos
Skip	- Fried food - Fried chicken - French fries, onion rings - Mayo, "special" sauce - "Value meals," which are too much food - Fountain sodas and milk shakes	- Fried noodles (with soups) - Fried rice - Anything deep fried: egg rolls and items that say General Tso's, Kung Pao, Moo Shu, or deep fried	-Pizzas with meat toppings - Alfredo sauces, cheesy dishes, and meat or sausage sauces - Veal scallopini or parmigiana dishes	- Huge plates of nachos topped with meat and cheese - Cheese dipping sauces or cheese dishes - Sour cream - Refried beans
Other Tips	- For sub sandwiches, "build" your own sandwich on whole wheat bread with turkey, roast beef, or ham; a small amount of cheese; and lots of veggies. - Order a "kids' meal" for a smaller portion. - Some places have low-fat ice cream – order a baby size portion if you want dessert.	- Order "No MSG," which is a form of salt. - If you take food home, add extra rice, noodles, and veggies to reduce the salt and fat. - Share meals or take some home, as portions of Chinese food can be huge.	- For your bread, ask for soft-tub margarine or olive oil, and use only a small amount. - If you're choosing pizza, go with a thin crust and order it "light on the cheese."	- If the restaurant offers free tortilla chips, put a small handful on a little plate and dip into salsa rather than a cheese sauce. - Ask for half the cheese or no cheese.

Can You Make Healthier Choices at Mini-Marts?

If you are a local trucker, you may find yourself visiting coffee shops or mini-marts for quick, cheap, and easy meals. What can you choose to keep calories, fat, and sodium in line? We have some tips "in store" for you.

Five mini-mart tips:

1. Look in the next section, "Think Before You Drink," for the best drink options.

2. Grabbing a sandwich? Look for mini-markets with submarine sandwiches so you can build your own healthy sandwich.

   - Choose turkey, grilled chicken, lean ham, or roast beef for your sub sandwich and load it with veggies.

   - For sandwich sauces, mustards and spices are safe. Go light on the mayo and other "special" sauces since dressings can add up fast.

3. For snack foods, take advantage of any "single serve" packs, or package them into small snack containers. Look for fruit/cheese/nut snack kits.

4. A serving of nuts is about one small handful. Portion this amount into a small container to avoid overdoing it.

5. Many mini-marts now have fresh fruit – grab a piece.

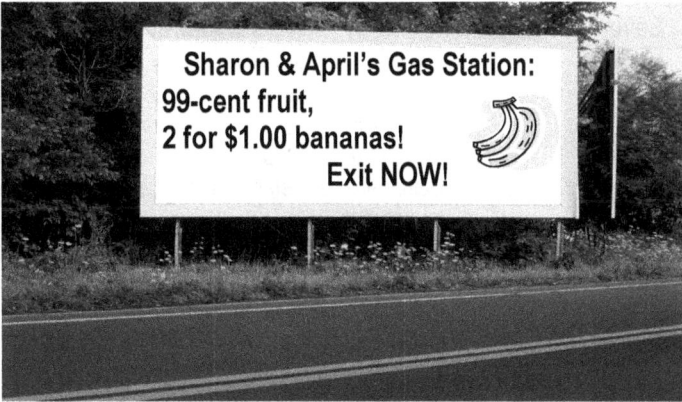

Think Before You Drink

We have talked a lot about choosing healthier foods when on the run. However, it is also important to think about your drinks. Many people forget about the calories and high amounts of sugar in drinks. Additionally, some research suggests that our brains do not detect that we have consumed anything when we get calories from drinks. Sweetened drinks are a great way to gain weight. So, what should you drink? Read the "Beverage Chart" on the next page for some suggestions.

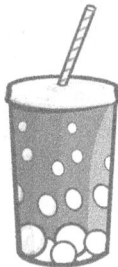

Beverage Chart	
Beverage:	**Tips & Information:**
Water and Teas	- Bottled water is a great choice, including calorie-free, flavored waters. (Remember to recycle bottles, or use a container from home for water.) - If you like teas, go for unsweetened or diet versions. Calorie-free sweeteners like Splenda® are OK in moderation.
Coffee	- Try coffee with low-fat milk or use just one creamer. - Try using only a small amount of sugar or calorie-free sweeteners like Splenda® if you need a sweetener. - For iced coffees: Ask for these to be made "skinny" (made with low-fat milk) with "no whip" (no whipped cream).
Juice	- Look for juices that say "100% juice," and keep your portion small – stick to only 8 ounces of juice per day. - Remember: Eating the fruit is better than drinking the juice since fruit has fiber – one glass of orange juice has half a gram of fiber. One orange has three grams of fiber. Eat the orange.
Soda, Carbonated Beverages, and Sweetened Drinks	- Sweetened drinks like soda, iced tea, lemonade, fruit punch, Sunny Delight® and Kool-Aid® are loaded with sugar and calories. - Avoid or limit these. Stick to one 12-ounce can per week, or switch to diet versions in moderation. - A typical can of soda has approximately 12 teaspoons of sugar.
Sports Drinks and Energy Drinks	- Choose the "light" or "Zero Calorie" versions. - Or, dilute sports drinks with half water or put in a container filled with lots of ice.
Alcoholic Beverages	- One glass of wine or beer has about 150 calories; so again, you will need to watch your portions. - Moderation is best: Limit yourself to one to two alcoholic beverages, and reconsider how often you drink.

Portion Control

Portion control is key. First, eat on a plate, not on a platter. When making choices:

- Eat a whole plate of salad with lots of fresh veggies and a drizzle of Italian or oil and vinegar-based salad dressing.
- Limit your bread to one or two pieces.
- Drink a big glass of water with ice and lemon.
- Make a MyPlate:
    - Keep protein foods to the size of a deck of cards or the size of your palm. Remember, protein foods include fish, meat, poultry, pork, or seafood.
    - Eat pasta or rice the size of your fist.
    - Fill the rest of your plate with vegetables and fruit.

Above all, eat with gusto! Enjoy each bite and really taste your food. If you don't like it, don't eat it. Once you are full, stop eating. You do not need to *clean your plate.*

References

1. Whitfield Jacobson PJ, Prawitz AD, Lukaszuk JM. Long-haul truck drivers want healthful meal options at truck-stop restaurants. *J Am Diet Assoc.* 2007;107(12):2125-2129.

Chapter 4:

Healthier Choices to Pack in Your Cab

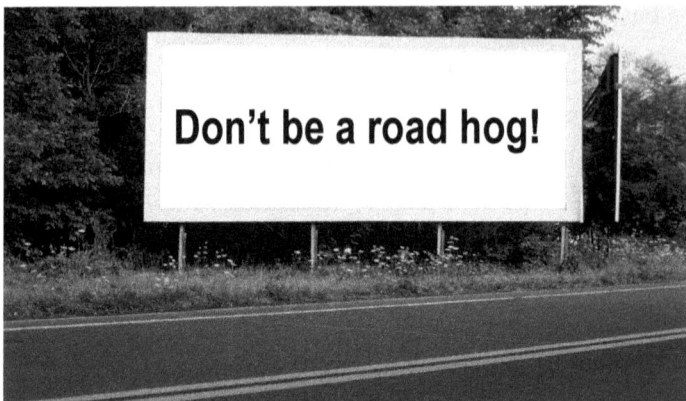

Eating away from home can be difficult if you do not have control over your food choices. Some fast food and convenience store items do not give you the right nutrition and energy you need to "keep on truckin'."

On the following pages are lists of healthier food choices to pack in your rig. Many do not require utensils, but if needed, pack plasticware. If you have a portable refrigerator or cooler, you have more healthy options available to you.

Be careful. Although these foods are packed with nutrients, remember to choose snack-size portions in small containers rather than eating food out of the original packages. Be cautious: Some snacks have two or more servings per bag, so portion these out. Keep only a few items in your cab at a time so you do not run the risk of eating out of boredom.

Rule of thumb: Check those labels. Per serving, look for:

- A snack with protein and fiber to feel full

- Less than 200 calories

- 5 grams of fat or less

- Less than 20 grams of carbohydrate if you have diabetes.

- If you have pre-diabetes or diabetes, choose sugar-free foods if available.

Healthier Food Choices to Pack in Your Rig:
Refrigerator or Cooler Needed:
-String cheese -Reduced fat cheese -Light cheese bites (such as Laughing Cow®) -Single-serving containers of cottage cheese -Low-fat milk -Yogurt -Portable yogurt such as GoGurt® -Drinkable yogurt smoothies or shots (less than 100 calories and 3 grams fat) -Healthy cold meat such as turkey, chicken, lean ham, or lean roast beef -Hard-boiled eggs -Any fresh fruit such as apples or grapes *Look for Farmers' Markets with local produce at some highway rest stops or roadside stands. -Baby carrots or other cut-up veggies such as cucumbers, celery or pepper strips -Low-fat dips, salsas, and hummus -Frozen edamame (shelled and thawed)

Healthier Food Choices to Pack in Your Rig:

No Refrigeration Needed:

-Whole grain bread, small tortilla wraps, small bagels, small homemade muffins
-Low sugar dry cereals such as Cheerios®, Wheaties®, Shredded wheat®, Chex cereals®, Kashi Seven Whole Grain Puffs or Flakes®, or oatmeal
-Nonfat dried milk (just add water)
-Low-fat granola bars, energy bars or cereal bars (less than150 calories and 3 grams fat)
-Pretzels or whole grain crackers such as Triscuits® or graham crackers
-Mini-bags of light microwaveable popcorn
-Baked potato chips
-Animal crackers
-Reduced sodium canned or aseptic boxed soups
-Canned beans
-Beef, turkey, or venison jerky (Note: Less than 300 mg sodium per serving)
-Dried fruit such as raisins, dried cranberries, or dried apricots
-Single-serving containers of fruit packed in light syrup, water or its own juice
-Bananas, apples, or pears
-6-ounce 100% fruit juice boxes (*Limit these to one box per day.)
-Bottled water
-Single-serving containers of gelatin (available with fruit or without)
-Single-serving containers of pudding (less than 100 calories and 3 grams fat)
-Peanut butter
-Chicken or tuna packed in water (in pouches or StarKist Lunch To-Go®)
-Canned salmon or crabmeat
-Nuts such as almonds, pecans or walnuts

Don't Drink Your Calories

Regular sodas, sweetened teas, energy or sports drinks, fruit drinks and 100% fruit juices, in excess, can load your body with unwanted sugar calories. And if you have diabetes or pre-diabetes, these drinks can wreak havoc on your blood sugars.

To stay hydrated and energized, stock your rig with these beverages:

- Water

- Calorie-free flavored water

- Diet soda

- Unsweetened teas

- Diluted 100% fruit juice (mix 4 ounces 100% fruit juice with lots of water)

- Purchased, ready-made smoothies (250 calories or less) or make your own smoothie: Using a blender or hand-held immersion blender, mix low-fat milk, banana, yogurt, and peanut butter. Blend in other fruit such as berries if available. If ice is available, blend in ice to make the smoothie frothy.

Appliances to Go

If you have access to electrical outlets, these appliances can help you pack a greater variety of healthy choices in your rig and allow you to do more cooking, when possible.

- Small refrigerator

- Microwave

- Crockpot

- Single serve blender with travel lid

- Hand-held immersion blender

Other Helpful Gadgets

- Personal portable ovens, such as HotLogic® Mini, and stoves, such as RoadPro®.

- Portable Grill

- Kitchen supplies: Can opener, Thermos, foil, saran wrap

Plan Ahead

Whether you decide to use convenience meals and snacks or cook your own meals, planning ahead of time is an important strategy. This ensures that you have all the foods and ingredients on hand so you do not end up relying on convenient store food. If you are on the road for extended weeks, stop at supermarkets or large convenience stores with large parking lots and seasonal farmer's markets at rest stops to re-stock your rig, especially with fresh fruits and vegetables.

Take advantage of the time when you are home to shop and prepare healthful foods that you can take on the road. Here are just a few ideas of foods that can be made ahead of time and then chilled and reheated:

- Grilled chicken or other lean meat
- Cooked pasta, noodles, or rice
- Fresh, cut-up veggies seasoned with herbs and olive oil, wrapped in foil, and grilled for 10 minutes.

And remember to use the convenient Truckers Grocery List in Appendix E (page 131) to help you select healthful foods for the road.

Chapter 5:

How to Lose Weight

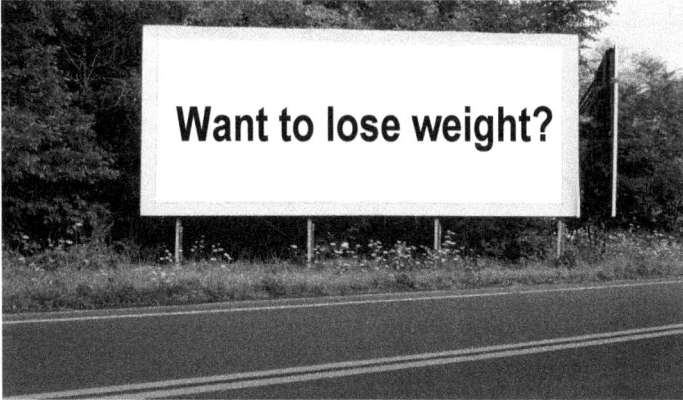

Losing weight is not easy for anyone. And it certainly doesn't help that your job includes a lot of sitting, little time for safe exercise, and the need for quick meals. In addition, you may, like many people, eat out of boredom instead of eating "mindfully."

While 60-75% of Americans are overweight or obese, it has been suggested that up to 90% of truck drivers are overweight or obese (1). The odds are stacked against you, but we can help.

How to Lose Weight

All foods have calories, and calories give you energy. If you eat more calories than your body needs, you will gain weight.

Additionally, if you eat past the feeling of fullness or eat when you are not hungry, you will likely gain weight.

If you normally drink three, 12-ounce sodas a day (which equals about 500 calories) and stop drinking the sodas all together, you will have decreased your calorie intake significantly, which would, in turn, lead to weight loss.

To lose weight, some people use the MyPlate as their guide, doing their best to make more nutritious choices and eat smaller portion sizes. Other people need more structure: recording everything they eat and drink or using an app for accountability. Either approach is OK; do what works for you.

* Note: See Appendix B for recommended websites and apps related to weight management.

Regardless of which weight loss method you choose, the basics of weight loss are eating fewer calories and exercising more. And if you want individualized help from a nutrition expert, find a Registered Dietitian Nutritionist in your area at: **EatRight.org**. (* Click "Find an Expert" at the top right of the webpage or at the very bottom of the page if you are using your smart phone.)

Eat Less

Wondering how you can eat less? Here, you will find a list of ideas for cutting back:

1. Eat "less" of the following when you have them, and make it "less often:"

- Hot dogs, fast food, chicken wings, fried foods
- Foods with cream sauces, gravies, and butter
- French fries, potato chips, other fried or fatty snacks
- Whole milk, eggs, mayonnaise, ice cream
- Cakes, cookies, donuts, pies
- Soda, sweetened iced tea, fruit juice, lemonade
- Beer, margaritas, excessive amounts of alcoholic beverages

Instead, save these foods for once in a while. You **can** eat these foods in moderation, thinking of them as special treats for once in a while. However, on a daily basis, choose the most nutritious options possible by using MyPlate as your guide.

2. Limit "play foods."

- Out of sight, out of mind: Keep sweets, treats, and snacks – "play foods" – for once in a while and stored away in the pantry or cupboard.

3. Eat breakfast.

- Believe it or not, eating a satisfying, MyPlate breakfast will help you stay full longer.

4. Keep snack foods stored away in the cupboard and fruit on the table.

- You will be more likely to grab a piece of fruit for a snack if it is right in front of you.

5. Keep your dinner items on the stovetop or counter instead of in front of you on the table.

- If you are still hungry, walk over for a small helping of seconds.

6. In the same way, put your snacks on a plate at home or in a baggie for work instead of eating out of the bag.

- By portioning out your snacks, you will eat much less.
- If you are at home and want more of your snack, you will actually have to move to get more.

7. Cut up raw veggies – or buy them already cut – and store them in food storage bags.

- Then, before work, you can pack a baggie or two for your shift.

8. Resist fast food as best you can.

- If you need to stop for fast food on occasion, you can order a more healthful option:
  Example: A plain hamburger or a grilled chicken sandwich without mayo, small fries, and a water – which is far healthier when compared to a "value" meal.

9. Eat smaller portions.

- Use smaller plates, bowls, and drinking glasses.

- Eat regularly scheduled meals and snacks to avoid extreme hunger, eating every four to five hours according to your hunger.

10. At restaurants:

- Do your best to order the most nutritious meal – one that is not fried. Choose an item that is grilled or baked, without added butter/sauces, and includes vegetables or a salad.

- You can share a meal or pack half of the meal in a takeout box if you have a cold pack or a refrigerator in your truck.

11. While eating, think about the following:

- Before eating, ask yourself: "Am I really hungry?"

- During the meal, ask yourself: "Am I still hungry?"

- Listen to your body: Eat when hungry, and stop when full.

- Do not skip meals, but don't graze all day long either.

- Eat something every four to five hours.

12. Try your best not to eat while doing other things.

- At home, get the television out of the kitchen.

- Enjoy eating in the company of others.

- Taste each bite of your food and take pleasure in it.

- Put away all distractions, including your phone.

13. Re-think your beverages.

- Stop drinking liquid sugars: Drinks like soda, lemonade, sweetened iced tea, fruit drinks, energy drinks, and even sports drinks are full of sugar which can cause you to *gain* weight.

- Did you know that juice – even 100% juice – has the same amount of sugar as sodas? Limit juice to 8 ounces a day or avoid it altogether.

- You may consume diet drinks in moderation. (In case you are wondering: Yes, diet drinks *do* have caffeine, unless they are labeled "caffeine-free.")

- Drink low-fat milk and save on calories. All milks contain the same amount of vitamins and minerals; the only difference between whole milk and low-fat milk is that low-fat milk is lower in calories and saturated fat.

- Drink lots of water. Water is the best beverage, and it will keep you hydrated. To give water flavor, squeeze in some lemon or orange.

Cut Down on Time in Front of Screens

Limit television, computer, and video game time to less than 10 hours per week. When viewing TV shows, know that a 30-minute show has 21 minutes of actual show time. The other nine minutes is commercials – time for you to get up and stretch, move, walk, march in place, do jumping jacks, and sit-ups and push-ups. Therefore, if you watch two hours of TV, you will actually have 36 minutes of commercial time to *exercise*.

Exercise More

Chapter 9 will focus on exercise and tips for you as a truck driver. The Office of Disease Prevention and Health Promotion recommends that adults ages 18 to 65 get at least 30 minutes of moderate intensity activity five days of the week (2). This exercise should get your heart pumping, and you should be sweating. Aim to get 10,000 steps in a day. To measure your steps, use your smart phone or wear an activity/step tracker.

Eat Mindfully

What does it mean to eat mindfully? It is a simple concept:

- Be aware while you are eating: Limit distractions by turning off the TV, your smart phone, and the computer.
- Eat when you are hungry, and stop when you are full. You do not have to clean your plate.
- It is better to listen to your body's signal of fullness than to worry about "wasting food."
- Take your time eating, taste your food, and really enjoy each bite.

- If you do not like something, stop eating it. It is not satisfying to eat something that does not taste good.
- Eat healthful, nutritious, and nourishing foods every day, but include all foods that you enjoy in moderation without guilt. "All foods can fit."

Some Other Tips for Healthy Eating

- Many people feel hungry several times a day rather than just three times a day. If this happens to you, don't be afraid to eat little meals and healthy snacks more often.
- Pay attention to your stomach and decide if you are really hungry.
- Be sure to eat a "breakfast meal" when you wake up. After a period of fasting, your body needs nourishment, and the breakfast meal can have a huge impact on your eating for the rest of the day.
- Eat at consistent times: If working through the night, consider eating a light meal before one AM, another light meal before sleep, and a larger "breakfast" meal when you wake (3).

If You Eat When You Are Bored

When truckers are bored, many eat, smoke, or chew tobacco to pass the time. Instead, try one of these activities:

- Talk to your driving assistant if you have one.
- Chew sugar-free gum.

- Crank up the music and sing your favorite tunes, if your driving assistant does not mind.
- Fidget and stretch your non-driving leg to move a bit.

Realistic, Safe Weight Loss

How much weight can you lose safely and realistically? It is recommended that you lose weight gradually – about one to two pounds per week. In addition, your new, healthier way of eating should not be a *diet*; instead, it should become a new way of living or a new habit for life.

Fad diets, on the other hand, promote quick weight loss; however, once you stop following the fad, you will re-gain the weight. You may even gain more weight back. When people lose weight, they may lose both fat and muscle. When they re-gain the weight, they may only gain back the fat. The muscle the dieter had before the fad diet may be lost, leaving the fad dieter with more body fat compared to before the diet.

Which diets are fad diets? Any diet that sounds too good to be true is probably a fad diet, like the high protein, low carbohydrate diets (where you can eat eggs and steak all day). Some other fads include miracle pills or dietary supplements that make big promises (commonly seen in magazine ads or on late night television infomercials) and exercise equipment that promises "spot reduction," among many others.

There are many websites that describe fads and their side effects. Some include:

- webmd.com (Search 'fad diets.')
- heart.org (Search 'fad diets.')

Becoming healthier is hard work and will take a lifelong commitment, so any quick fix for weight loss should make you suspicious. What advice is best? Take one day at a time, make the best health decisions possible, and have friends or family support you. All foods can fit, so if you eat something less nutritious, you haven't blown it. Think positively and give healthy eating and exercise your best effort. You can do it!

References

1. Sieber WK, Robinson CF, Birdsey J, Chen GX, Hitchcock EM, Lincoln JE. Obesity and other risk factors: The National Survey of U.S. long-haul truck driver health and injury. *Am J Ind Med.* (2014);57(6):615-626.

2. Office of Disease Prevention and Health Promotion. Physical Activity. Available at: https://health.gov/paguidelines. Accessed May 13, 2019.

3. Sawyer-Morse MK. Lunch at midnight: The impact of shift work on health. *Today's Dietitian,* 2006;8(6):55-56.

Chapter 6: How to Lower Blood Cholesterol, Triglycerides, and Blood Pressure

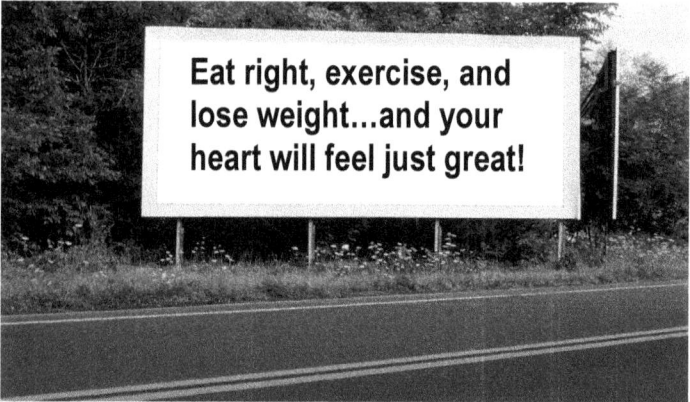

Eat right, exercise, and lose weight...and your heart will feel just great!

Do you have high cholesterol? Have you been told you have high triglycerides? Is your blood pressure too high? If you have answered "yes" to any of these questions, this chapter can provide you with some tips to improve your "numbers." Not sure what all these terms mean? We will teach you here, so read on.

All about Cholesterol

Cholesterol is waxy, sticky fat in our blood. Our bodies need some cholesterol to build cells and make hormones, but too much cholesterol can lead to heart disease.

- **Where does cholesterol come from?** We make some cholesterol in our bodies, and we also get cholesterol from animal foods like beef, pork, organ meats, fish, eggs, high-fat dairy foods, and poultry. Foods high in <u>saturated fats</u> and <u>trans fats</u> also contribute to cholesterol problems.

- **What are saturated fats?** Saturated fats come from animal food sources such as fatty meats, bacon, sausage, poultry skin, organ meats, whole milk, butter, and cheese. There are a few plant sources of saturated fat, which include coconut oil, palm oil, palm kernel oil, and cocoa butter found in chocolate.

- **What are trans fats?** Trans fats are chemically changed ("partially hydrogenated") fats, initially manufactured to add to foods to keep them fresh longer. Trans fats can be found in stick margarine, fast foods, fried foods, doughnuts, French fries, baked goods, and many packaged items. Look out for "trans fat" on the label.

- **Diets that are too high in saturated fat and trans fat raise "bad" cholesterol**, which can increase your risk of heart disease.

- **When it comes to saturated fats, <u>eat less.</u>** You can do this by eating more poultry, fish, and game meat instead of red meat and by switching to low-fat dairy foods. Keep red meats to twice a week or less.

- **<u>Avoid</u> trans fat:** Look on food labels for "0 grams trans fat."

- **However,** "trans fat free" foods may still be high in saturated fat: Become a careful label reader, looking for low saturated *and* trans fats.

Better Fats

"Better" fats are those that are <u>unsaturated</u>. These fats include mono<u>unsaturated</u> fats and poly<u>unsaturated</u> fats. These fats are better because they can lower your risk of heart disease.

- **Monounsaturated fats** include olive oil, canola oil, peanut oil, avocados, and nuts.
    - Replace your current oils with olive, canola, or peanut oil.
- **Polyunsaturated fats** include all of the other vegetable oils (like soybean, corn, safflower, and sesame oil) and also the heart healthy, "omega-3 fatty acids."
    - Instead of butter, switch to a soft-tub margarine, preferably one that is "light."
    - Avoid stick margarine, a source of trans fat.
- **Omega-3 fatty acids** come from fatty fish like salmon, trout, and tuna or from "fish oil supplements," as they may lower the risk of heart disease and prevent inflammation.
    - Eat fatty fish like salmon, trout, or tuna at least twice a week or more.

Fat is Still Fat: Moderation is Key

Eat less saturated fat, try to avoid trans fats, and choose unsaturated fats. But does that mean you can deep-fry daily in olive oil? Not so. Fat is still fat, and it is higher in calories than protein or carbohydrates. Plain and simple: You do need some fat, but use it in moderation. (For more information on the different types of fats, see: Heart.org.)

What Are the Different Types of Cholesterol and What Should My Numbers Be?

In a laboratory test for cholesterol or a "lipid profile," you will likely see the following four measurements for cholesterol. Read on for a description of each term, the number you should aim for, and in boxes, recommendations for improving each based on the guidelines of the American Heart Association (1). For more information, see: Heart.org.

1. **Total Cholesterol** – is a measurement of a combination of the types of cholesterol circulating in your blood.

   Where should your Total Cholesterol be?

   - Shoot for less than 200 milligrams per deciliter.
   - A high cholesterol level can increase your risk of heart attack and stroke. Your doctor will also take into account other risk factors such as age, family history, smoking, and high blood pressure.
   - Talk to your doctor about your cholesterol and how your numbers impact your overall risk for heart disease.

IF YOU ARE TOLD YOUR TOTAL CHOLESTEROL IS TOO HIGH:

- Talk to your doctor about treatment options.
- Eat healthy foods, like those we mention in this book.
- Choose less animal fats like butter, whole milk, and red meats.
- Avoid trans fats.
- Eat more fiber, found in fruits, vegetables, beans/legumes, and whole grains.
- Exercise regularly.
- Quit smoking.
- Lose weight.
- You may need medication.
- Ask your doctor how often you should have your cholesterol rechecked.

---

2. **HDL** – is a measurement of your high-density lipoprotein (HDL) levels or "good" cholesterol. Think of it this way: HDL should be **High**. HDL removes cholesterol build-up from your body.

Where should your HDL be?

- Aim for an HDL number over 40.
- A high level of HDL can protect you against heart attack and stroke.
- Talk to your doctor about your HDL and how your numbers impact your overall risk for heart disease.

> ### *IF YOU ARE TOLD YOUR HDL IS TOO LOW:*
>
> - Exercise every day for at least 30 minutes.
> - Lose weight.
> - Quit smoking.
> - Eat foods with better fats such as salmon, seafood, tuna, and olive or canola oils.
> - Cut out trans fats.

3. **LDL** – is a measurement of your low-density lipoprotein (LDL) levels or "bad" cholesterol and is linked with heart disease. The lower your LDL, the better. Think of it this way: LDL should be **L**ow. Too much LDL can build up inside your arteries.

Where should your LDL be?

- Aim for an LDL less than 100. A high LDL level can increase your risk of heart attack and stroke.
- Talk to your doctor about your LDL and how your numbers impact your overall risk for heart disease.

> ### *IF YOU ARE TOLD YOUR LDL IS TOO HIGH:*
>
> - Eat less total fat, less saturated fat (from animal foods), and less trans fats.
> - Lose weight.
> - Eat high-fiber foods and plenty of soluble fiber, found in fresh fruits, vegetables, and whole grains.
> - You may need medication.

4. **Triglycerides** – are another type of blood fat. They come from food and your body makes them.

Where should your Triglycerides be?

- Aim for a triglyceride number less than 150. A high triglyceride level can increase your risk of heart attack and stroke.

- Talk to your doctor about your triglycerides and how your numbers impact your overall risk for heart disease.

IF YOU ARE TOLD YOUR TRIGLYCERIDES ARE TOO HIGH:

- Lose weight and eat healthy foods, like those we mention in this book.
- Eat less saturated and trans fats and more fiber.
- Limit sugary beverages and sweets.
- Limit alcohol to 1 drink a day for women and 2 drinks a day for men.
- Begin exercising.
- Quit smoking.
- If you have diabetes, improve your blood sugars (See Chapter 7).
- You may need medication or fish oil supplements.

All about Blood Pressure

Sometimes, people do not even know they have high blood pressure since there are often no symptoms (2). So why is it so important to know your blood pressure? Undetected and untreated high blood pressure can lead to stroke, heart attack, heart failure, or kidney failure. So, get your numbers checked!

> ***The normal value for blood pressure is less than 120/80 mmHg.***
>
> ****Check with your doctor for your individual blood pressure goals.***

If you do have high blood pressure, the American Heart Association recommends making the following diet and lifestyle changes (3):

- Reduce the fat in your diet (particularly saturated or animal fats and trans fats).
- Eat less salt and cut down on high sodium foods.
- Eat potassium-rich foods (if allowed; some people with kidney problems need to restrict potassium).
- Change your lifestyle by losing weight and getting regular physical activity. Manage stress.
- Quit smoking to reduce your overall risk for heart attack and stroke.
- Reduce the amount of alcohol you drink.
- Take medications to control high blood pressure if prescribed by your doctor.

First, Let's Talk about Eating Less Sodium

Who needs to eat less sodium? The truth is: All Americans need less sodium, and those with high blood pressure need to be extra careful with salty foods to help prevent heart attack, stroke, or kidney problems. So, what are some guidelines for eating a lower salt diet? Here are three tips:

1. *Throw out the salt shaker.*

- We're serious: Get the salt shaker off the table.
- Instead of salt, use other seasonings like onion powder, garlic powder, pepper, Mrs. Dash®, and other herbs and spices.
- You can also be creative with lemon, herbs, hot sauce, and liquid smoke to flavor foods.
- Choose reduced sodium soy sauce and use smaller quantities.
- Be aware that "salt substitutes" usually replace sodium with potassium, which you may need to restrict. Be sure to check with your doctor first about these products.

2. *Read labels.*

- Look for less than 140 mg sodium per serving.
- Aim for no more than 2,300 mg sodium per day, with an ideal limit of no more than 1,500 mg a day for most adults.
- Choose foods that say "low sodium."
- But be careful with those that say "reduced sodium," as these may still be high in salt. If you use "reduced sodium" foods, stick to the serving size on the label.

3. *Eat fresh, unprocessed foods and low sodium products.*

- Choose fresh foods and unprocessed, natural meats.

- Choose fresh or frozen vegetables instead of the canned varieties, and use frozen vegetables that don't have sauce added. If using canned, choose "no salt added."

- Limit frozen meals, which may be too salty. Look for less than 500 mg sodium per meal.

- Avoid cured, processed, or canned meats like deli meats, Spam®, sausage, bacon, hot dogs, and American cheese, which are extremely high in salt. Check at the deli to see if low salt deli meats and cheese are available.

- Take-out, fast foods, and restaurant foods most always have high amounts of sodium. You can ask for less salt when ordering and choose not to use salt at the table.

- Watch the sodium content of snack foods. Even the healthy types may be loaded with salt.

- Remember: With "reduced" sodium foods, check the label with a watchful eye. Choose foods with less than 140 mg sodium.

Now Let's Talk about Adding More Potassium to Your Diet

- Lowering salt intake and adding potassium-rich foods can help lower your blood pressure.

- Fruits, vegetables, whole grain foods, and low-fat dairy foods provide potassium.

- High potassium fruits and vegetables include bananas, oranges, potatoes, spinach, and tomatoes.
- The DASH (Dietary Approaches to Stop Hypertension) Diet can help you add potassium and other important nutrients to your diet (4).

For More Information

There are other ways to lower blood pressure such as decreasing fat, exercising, losing weight, quitting smoking, and taking medication. We give recommendations on "how to" make these changes throughout this book

References

1. American Heart Association Web site. What your cholesterol levels mean. Available at: heart.org. Accessed September 9, 2018.
2. American Heart Association Web site. High blood pressure. Available at: heart.org. Accessed September 9, 2018.
3. American Heart Association Web site. Changes you can make to manage high blood pressure. Available at: heart.org. Accessed September 9, 2018.
4. The DASH Diet Eating Plan. Available at: dashdiet.org. Accessed September 9, 2018.

Chapter 7: Pre-Diabetes and Diabetes:
How to Manage Your Blood Sugar

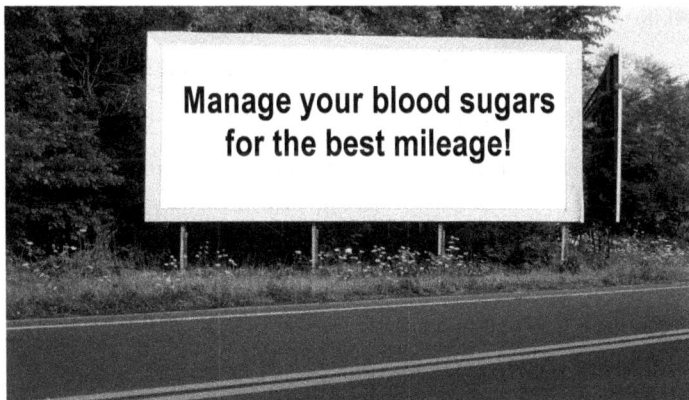

As we age, we may start to see increases in our blood sugar (glucose). If your doctor does blood work and finds your glucose levels are above the normal range, you may be diagnosed with pre-diabetes or Type 2 diabetes.

Normally, when you eat, your body breaks the food down into blood sugar. As you are making blood sugar, your pancreas puts out a hormone called insulin to help move the sugar from your blood into your cells. Once in the cells, the blood sugar turns into energy.

Diabetes is a disease in which your body may not make enough insulin or your cells ignore the insulin. When this happens, the blood sugar cannot move into the cells and starts to build up in your blood. Your cells then become starved for energy.

Pre-diabetes often develops before actual diabetes. You can have pre-diabetes if your blood sugar levels are higher than normal, but not yet high enough to be diagnosed with diabetes.

Before a meal (also called fasting), your blood sugar should be less than 100 milligrams/deciliter (mg/dl). If your fasting blood sugar is between 100 and 125 mg/dl, you have pre-diabetes. If your fasting blood sugar is greater than 126 mg/dl, you have diabetes. Your doctor may do other blood tests to confirm the diagnosis of either pre-diabetes or diabetes.

Diabetes is a disease that you should take seriously. If left untreated, high blood sugar levels can eventually lead to damage to your eyes, heart, kidneys, and nerves, especially in your feet – the damage from diabetes can impact your body from "head to toe."

Several factors can put you at risk for having diabetes:
- age 45 or older
- a family history of diabetes
- high blood pressure: above 140 over 90
- triglycerides of 250 or higher
- low HDL ("good") cholesterol: less than 35
- diabetes when pregnant/delivered a large baby (over 9 lbs.)
- women with polycystic ovary syndrome (PCOS)
- overweight or obese
- not physically active on a regular basis.

You are also at higher risk if you are a member of any of these ethnic groups: Black or African-American, Latino, Alaska Native or American Indian, Asian American, and Native Hawaiian or other Pacific Islander. To learn about your risk for diabetes, visit the American Diabetes Association website (diabetes.org) and complete the Diabetes Risk Test.

Treatment for Diabetes

If you are diagnosed with pre-diabetes or diabetes, the good news is both conditions can be treated especially if caught early. And you can prevent many of the "head to toe" complications if you keep your blood sugars under good control.

You may be able to manage your pre-diabetes with just diet and exercise. Sometimes diabetes may warrant taking medication, especially if your blood sugars are abnormally high. But diet and exercise will still play an important role in controlling blood sugars.

Your doctor may suggest you see a registered dietitian nutritionist (RDN) or certified diabetes educator (CDE) who can create an eating and exercise plan geared toward your lifestyle to help manage your blood sugars. You may also learn how to take your blood sugars using a special meter called a glucometer. If you are on the road following a hectic work and eating schedule, it would be especially helpful for you to monitor your blood sugars with your glucometer.

Nutrition Tips for Pre-Diabetes and Diabetes

You can follow the same nutrition guidelines if you have pre-diabetes or diabetes. Eating well with either does not mean following a strict or special diet. It does mean eating healthy by following these guidelines:

- **Choose balanced meals.** Include a variety of foods in your diet. This includes carbohydrates which are grains, fruit, milk, yogurt and vegetables; protein which are meat and meat substitutes; and healthy fats such as olive and canola oils, tub margarines, and nuts. For good blood sugar control, include each of those nutrients (carbohydrate, protein, and fat) at each meal and snack.

- **Avoid skipping meals.** This can cause abnormal increases or decreases in your blood sugars. Try to eat every four to five hours and keep meal times around the same time each day. If you are going to have long delays between meals due to your busy work schedule, then plan a healthy snack with protein plus carbohydrate to hold you over to the next meal.

- **Be consistent with the size of your meals.** The more food you eat, the more blood sugar you will make. If meal sizes vary too much every day, your blood sugars will be less stable. These wide swings in blood sugar mean your diabetes is poorly controlled and can eventually lead to those "head to toe" complications.

- **Limit foods high in sugar.** These include all types of sweets like cake, pie, cookies, ice cream, and candy. Certain beverages are very high in sugar such as regular sodas, sweetened tea, fruit drinks, fruit juices, and energy drinks. Look for sugar-free foods and beverages made with sugar-substitutes like Splenda®, Sweet and Low®, or Truvia®, sugar-free gelatin, diet sodas, unsweetened tea or coffee, and some flavored waters.

- **Eat healthier fats and less of them.** With diabetes, you have a greater risk of heart disease and strokes. Saturated fats make your body more resistant to your insulin. Eating moderate amounts of healthier fats will protect your heart and help you manage your weight. Choose:
  - Fish, chicken and turkey with skin removed, and lean cuts of red meat. Trim fat from meats before cooking. Bake, broil, grill, roast or microwave food, rather than frying.
  - Fatty fish such as salmon, trout, or tuna at least twice a week.
  - Small amounts of tub margarine and vegetable oils such as olive oil. When available, choose light versions of tub margarine, salad dressings and mayonnaise.
  - Dairy products with less fat such as low-fat milk and yogurt, low-fat or reduced fat cheese, and low-fat (and low sugar) ice cream and frozen yogurt.

- **If you drink alcohol, consume it in moderation** – one drink a day for women, and no more than two drinks a day for men. It is best to drink with a meal or snack to avoid extreme blood sugar fluctuations or low blood sugars.

Putting It All Together

Now let's put it all together. Based on our suggestions in this chapter, here is a sample menu that includes all the healthy diet recommendations for people with diabetes. Rather than following this menu exactly, check out how we have incorporated whole grains, fruits, vegetables, low-fat dairy, and healthy meats. See the sample menu on the next page, and try to create a similar menu for yourself each day.

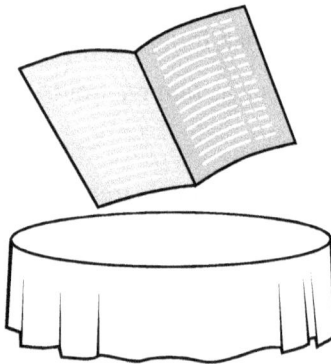

Sample Menu for People with Diabetes
Breakfast idea: Cereal such as Wheaties® or oatmeal with low-fat milk Whole wheat toast with peanut butter or another nut butter Fresh fruit or unsweetened canned fruit
Lunch idea: Turkey sandwich made with 2 pieces whole grain bread, small stack of sliced turkey, provolone, lettuce, tomato, light mayo Fresh fruit or unsweetened canned fruit Cut peppers, cucumbers, or baby carrots
Dinner idea: Broiled or baked fish or chicken Small baked potato or sweet potato with soft-tub margarine Steamed vegetables Small frozen yogurt
Snack idea: 6 Saltines with peanut butter Small apple

Follow the "diabetes plate method" when designing your meals. Limit carbohydrates and protein to one quarter each of a small plate, and fill the other half of the plate with non-starchy vegetables.

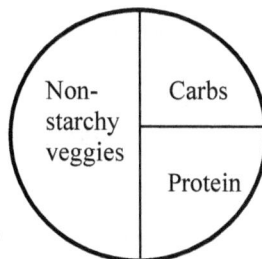

References

1. American Diabetes Association. Diabetes.org. Accessed February 2, 2018.

Chapter 8:

How to Stay Energized

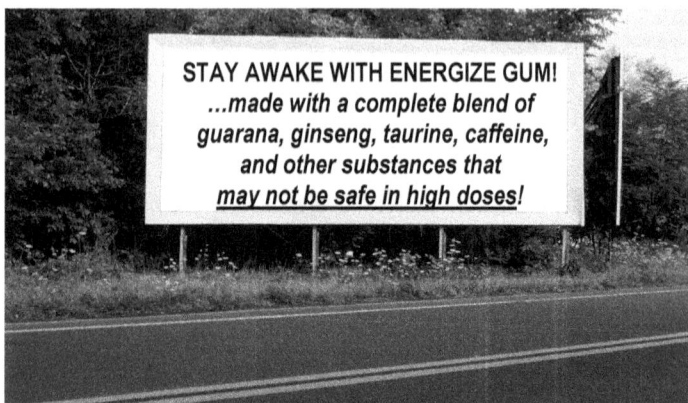

STAY AWAKE WITH ENERGIZE GUM!
...*made with a complete blend of guarana, ginseng, taurine, caffeine, and other substances that may not be safe in high doses!*

Whether you choose Red Bull®, Mountain Dew®, coffee, energy pills or bars, or something else, we know you need to stay awake to do your job. Therefore, the point of this chapter is to provide you with *healthier* ways to stay awake. Truth is: There are a lot of questionable products out there...we will help you decipher the safe from the unsafe.

Harmful Energizing Habits

First and foremost, let's explore which energy habits may be harmful to your health:

- **Smoking or chewing tobacco to stay awake** – The negative effects of tobacco are well known. See chapter 10 for more on quitting and eating right when trying to quit.

- **Eating to stay awake** – Eating when you are **not** hungry can lead to weight and heart problems. Eat only when you are hungry and stop when you are full.

- **Drinking energy drinks that have many herbals** – Herbals can be dangerous, plain and simple. (Read on for more information on herbs that are commonly found in energy drinks.)

- **Drinking caffeine or energy drinks that have calories** – Just like soda, any energy drink that has calories can lead to weight gain. Be aware of calories as you are choosing an energy aid.

- **Eating energy bars or foods** – Much the same as energy drinks, the extra calories in "energy" foods can lead to weight gain if you are consuming too much or eating when not hungry.

- **Using energy pills or gums** – While these are plentiful at gas stations and truck stops, know that energy pills or dietary supplements can be downright dangerous.

Common Herbals/Dietary Supplements Found in "Energy" Products

Look on the back of any "energy" products such as drinks, gums, gels, foods, and bars, and you will likely see any of the following combination of these herbals/dietary supplements: guarana, ginseng, taurine, and caffeine.

Guarana

Guarana is a rich source of caffeine that contains many other compounds. Very few studies have examined guarana alone; however, side effects do include irritability, heart palpitations, anxiety, and other central nervous system effects (1). Because of the potential for negative impacts on the central nervous system, many health authorities recommend avoiding guarana. Talk to your doctor or dietitian if you want more information or if you have any questions about guarana.

Ginseng

Ginseng is a slow growing plant that people use for many different reasons; however, there is not strong scientific evidence to prove significant benefits (2). When used at recommended doses, ginseng appears to be well tolerated with serious side effects being rare (2). For recommended doses, safety information, and drug interactions, visit: webmd.com/vitamins, and search 'ginseng.'

Taurine

Taurine is an amino acid (a building block of protein) in the body that we get from eating animal foods. While energy drink makers claim that taurine "helps flush toxins out of the body," the truth is: Taurine does not contain any special properties to boost energy (3).

Caffeine

Last but definitely not least: Caffeine is commonly added to many drinks and products and can be a powerful tool for energy and staying awake. The energizing effects of caffeine are seen within 15 minutes to two hours; although, those who consume it regularly may notice a lessening of its energizing effects over time (4).

What Caffeine Does to the Body

Caffeine has many effects on the body, both positive and negative. Many times, the effects of caffeine depend on the dose and on the person.

- **Some Positive Effects of Caffeine:** Caffeine increases alertness and can help with energy and physical performance. People who use caffeine report that they have more energy, are more alert, and have fewer headaches (4).

- **Some Negative Effects of Caffeine:** High amounts of caffeine affect sleep and can cause heartburn, restlessness, and anxiety (4). For women, a high caffeine intake can also lead to infertility and possibly miscarriage or birth defects; so, women should not consume more than 200 mg of caffeine per day, about 8 to 16 ounces of coffee (depending on the type), when trying to conceive or when pregnant (5, 6).

Many Truck Drivers NEED Coffee: Healthier Caffeine Use

- Consume moderate amounts of coffee – try sticking to three, eight-ounce cups or less per day (as long as you are not pregnant or attempting pregnancy).
- Drink coffee early in your shift so it won't affect your sleep, then switch to decaffeinated or caffeine-free versions of drinks – preferably unsweetened, sugar-free drinks.
- Instead of regular drinks with caffeine, choose diet drinks.
- Make healthier coffee: If you use cream, switch to 1% or fat-free milk, or try low-fat or fat-free half and half. Or, only put one creamer in your coffee. If you sweeten, try a sugar-free sweetener like Splenda® or Truvia®, or use less sugar (only one or two teaspoons per cup).

Energy Drinks, Pills, and Dietary Supplements

Do you take energy drinks, herbal, or nutritional supplements to stay awake, work harder, or increase your energy and strength? Be careful: These supplements may be *dangerous*!

According to the U. S. Food and Drug Administration (FDA), "dietary supplements include such ingredients as vitamins, minerals, herbs, amino acids, and enzymes. Dietary supplements are marketed in forms such as tablets, capsules, softgels, gelcaps, powders, and liquids" (7). Dietary supplements can come in many different forms and can contain vitamins, minerals, herbs or other botanicals, amino acids, and substances such as enzymes or even organ tissues (7).

According to the U.S. FDA, the Dietary Supplement Health and Education Act of 1994 places dietary supplements under the general umbrella of "foods," not drugs, and requires that every supplement be labeled a dietary supplement (7). As "foods" rather than medications, the U.S. FDA states:

> "FDA is not authorized to review dietary supplement products for safety and effectiveness **before they are marketed**. The manufacturers and distributors of dietary supplements are responsible for making sure their products are safe before they go to market. If a serious problem associated with a dietary supplement occurs, manufacturers must report it to FDA as an adverse event. FDA can take dietary supplements off the market if they are found to be unsafe or if the claims on the products are false and misleading" (8).

What does all this mean?

The manufacturer, *not the FDA*, is responsible for ensuring the supplement is safe *before* marketing. FDA doesn't get involved until after it is sold and *after* people take it and get sick from it. Only then is it deemed unsafe.

Since there is no monitoring of the dietary supplement industry as companies market and sell their dietary supplements, there are several problems that may arise:

- The supplements you take may not even contain what they are supposed to contain.
- The supplements you take may contain "fillers" and less of the active ingredient than they are supposed to contain.

- The supplements you take may be tainted by other substances.
- The supplements you take may have dangerous side effects.
- Do you take prescribed medications? Some herbals and dietary supplements may interact with your medications, leading to potentially dangerous side effects or even death.

What should you do about your current dietary supplements and herbals regimen? Talk with your doctor, pharmacist, or registered dietitian nutritionist about the supplements you are taking. Ask for their input, and heed their advice when it comes to dangerous supplement-medicine interactions. If in doubt, throw them out. And remember the following saying: "If it sounds too good to be true, it probably is."

If you choose to take a dietary supplement, follow these guidelines:

- Choose supplements made by better-known manufacturers.
- Check the label for adverse reactions.
- Take only one new product at a time.
- Start with the recommended dose or less than the recommended dose.
- Give your doctor a list of all the supplements you take.

Getting Energized: What to Do Instead of Eating When You Are Sleepy

Just as when truckers are bored, when truckers are sleepy, they may eat, smoke, or chew tobacco to stay awake. Try one of these activities instead:

- Talk to someone or talk out loud.
- Chew sugar-free gum.
- Crank up the music and sing to your favorite tunes.
- Tap your non-driving foot or leg.
- Take a break.
- Turn on the air conditioning (if your truck has it – otherwise, open a window).

When to Eat, What to Eat

If working overnight, try to eat a light meal before 1:00 AM, another light meal before sleeping, and your main meal after sleeping (9). For alertness, have small snacks containing protein in between meals. Protein-rich snacks include: string cheese, nuts, low-fat beef jerky, or turkey, chicken, lean beef, or reduced sodium ham or other sliced meats.

It is also helpful to eat meats/protein at the beginning of your shift to increase alertness, and then switch to carbohydrate snacks (fruit, starches, breads, cereals, low-fat snack foods) at the end of your shift (9). And most importantly, take a meal break at work.

Getting Energized: Taking a Break for a Nap

A 20-minute nap alone can give you a four-hour boost in alertness and productivity (9). If you have a driving partner or assistant or have time on your shift to take breaks, do so.

Other Ways to Stay Energized

There are other ways to stay energized, such as drinking enough fluids so you don't get dehydrated and exercising. Exercising and making the conscious choice to move are very important parts of a healthy lifestyle. Exercise is fully discussed in chapter 9. There are many ways to exercise without setting time aside for exercise alone:

Do you watch TV?

Did you know that each 30-minute segment of TV has approximately 21 minutes of "show" and nine minutes of commercials? If you watch two hours of TV each day, you can therefore use about 36 minutes of commercials to *move*. What can you do during commercials – or during the entire time you watch TV?

- Do sit-ups, push-ups, or jumping jacks during commercials.
- Walk in place or jog around your living room for each commercial.
- Lift dumbbells or use thera-bands for an entire 30-minute show.

- At home, put a treadmill or exercise machine in your TV room and walk on it during your favorite show.
- Do anything that involves movement, and this counts as exercise – all while watching your favorite shows.

Want to know something NEAT?

NEAT stands for Non-Exercise Activity Thermogenesis. This technical term for times when you are not "exercising" but still moving includes these actions:

- crossing your legs
- keeping good posture
- fidgeting your legs or hands and tapping your toes
- walking from a far-away parking spot to the store – or walking to the store and not taking the car
- taking the stairs instead of the elevator
- standing instead of sitting

Why move more or allow for some NEAT in your body?

Those people who move more or allow for more NEAT to occur in the body tend not to gain weight (10). So, do more of the things listed above, stand up more, and make an effort to move throughout your day.

References

1. Pittler MH, Schmidt K, Ernst E. Adverse events of herbal food supplements for body weight reduction: Systematic review. *Int J Obes Relat Metab Disord.* 2005;6:93-111.

2. U. S. National Library of Medicine & National Institutes of Health. Ginseng. Available at: nccih.nih.gov/health Accessed May 13, 2019.

3. Zamora D. Energy for sale: Energy products abound: in drinks, herbs, bars, and even goo. But do they do anything? Available at: webmd.com. Accessed May 13, 2019.

4. Cappelletti S, Piacentino D, Sani G, Aromatario M. Caffeine: Cognitive and Physical Performance Enhancer or Psychoactive Drug? *Current Neuropharmacology.* 2015;13:71-88.

5. Nisenblat V, Norman R. The effects of caffeine on reproductive outcomes in women. Available at: UpToDate®. Accessed June 14, 2019.

6. Krause's Food & the Nutrition Care Process, 14th ed., 2017.

7. U. S. Food and Drug Administration. Backgrounder on the Final Rule for Current Good Manufacturing Practices (CGMPs) for Dietary Supplements. Available at: FDA.gov. Accessed May 13, 2019.

8. U. S. Food and Drug Administration. Information for consumers: What You Need to Know about Dietary Supplements. Available at: FDA.gov. Accessed May 13, 2019.

9. Sawyer-Morse MK. Lunch at midnight: The impact of shift work on health. *Today's Dietitian,* 2006;8(6):55-56.

10. Levine JA, Eberhardt NL, Jensen MD. Role of nonexercise activity thermogenesis in resistance in fat gain in humans. *Science,* 1999;283:212-215.

Chapter 9:

Physical Activity

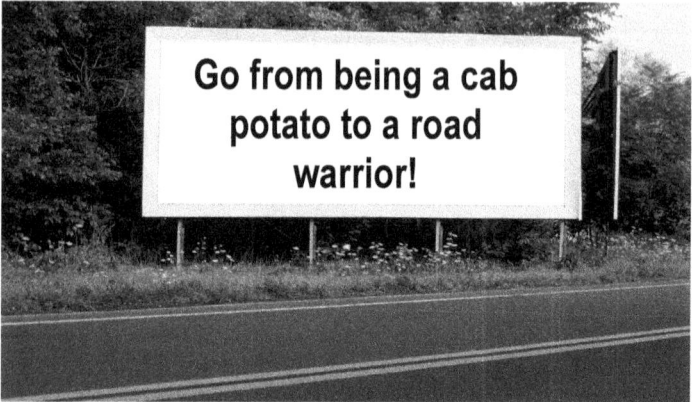

Go from being a cab potato to a road warrior!

Physical activity is so important for maintaining our health, but truck drivers have difficulty fitting it into their busy driving schedules. So, like many professions with long work hours, you just have to get creative about being physically active.

Once you make the commitment to move more, you will see the benefits of being more physically fit. The benefits of exercise include:

- keeps you energized so you are more alert while driving
- improves your sleep habits
- helps you burn calories more efficiently so you can lose or manage your weight
- maintains muscle strength to help with lifting
- prevents falls
- improves blood pressure

- decreases your "bad" cholesterol level and raises your "good" cholesterol level in your blood to prevent heart disease; lowers triglyceride levels in your blood to prevent strokes
- lowers blood sugars to help manage pre-diabetes and diabetes
- reduces depression
- may prevent some cancers such as colon and breast cancers

The easy part is admitting you need more physical activity, but the hard part is actually doing it when you do not have control over your busy schedule. If you make physical activity a priority and gradually build it into your schedule, you will be successful at becoming more active.

Caution: Before starting any increase in physical activity, be sure to have a check-up with your doctor. This is especially important if you have not been physically active on a regular basis. With any exercise, start out slowly and work your way up to a higher level.

Follow the "10 – 4" Rule

To go from being a cab potato to a road warrior, you just need a few simple props:

- Comfortable sneakers
- Hand weights (dumbbells)
- Your rig

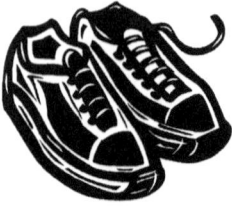 + 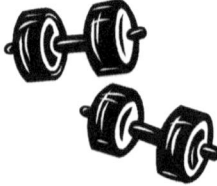 +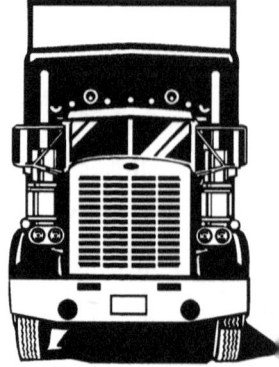

And then follow the "10 – 4 Rule":

- Wearing comfortable *sneakers*, do aerobic or heart and lung strengthening activity such as brief walking or jogging at least 4 times a day. Each session need only be 10 minutes in length.
- Lift *hand weights* 10 times (repetitions) to build muscle.
- You can use *your rig* if needed for your physical activity program.

The more you repeat the 10 – 4 Rule, the more physically fit you will become and the more health benefits you will see. Here are simple ways to apply the 10 – 4 Rule:

Muscle Building

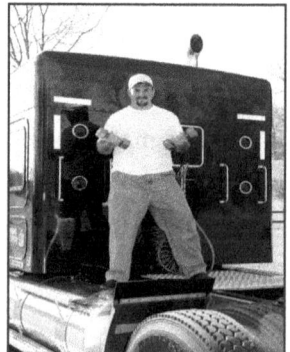

- Keep hand weights (dumbbells) in your rig. Do 10 repetitions of each: overhead press, triceps extensions, and biceps curls (see photo, right).

Rest and then do another round of each. If you cannot carry extra weight in your rig, then purchase Therabands® (theraband.com) to do your muscle building exercises. (For descriptions of these exercises, see Appendix B for helpful websites.)

- Do push ups while leaning against your rig (see photo, right).
  Face your rig with space between your body and the rig. Lean forward and place your palms flat against the rig at shoulder height and width apart. Slowly bend your elbows as you lower your upper body toward the rig keeping your feet flat on the ground. First do 10 reps with hands shoulder width apart to target your chest muscles, then move your hands to touching to work your triceps. Rest one to two minutes between each set of 10 reps.

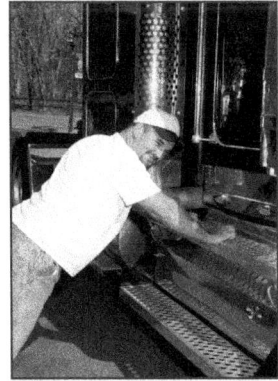

- While driving, suck in your abdominal muscles toward your spine, then breathe out and release. Do 10 repetitions, rest and repeat. Sit up straight and squeeze your buttocks, holding for as long as you can, about 10 seconds. Release, and repeat another four times.

- Sit up straight and place your feet flat on the floor. Press down with your toes and slowly lift your heels as high as they will go. Hold for 5 seconds, then lower your heels back down. Next, lift your toes off the floor, pressing down with your heel, until you feel the stretch. Hold for a few seconds, and lower your toes back down. Repeat, alternating heels and toes, 4 more times.

Heart and Lung Strengthening

- Walk just a total of 10 minutes at truck stops each time you take a break. If you park your rig farther away from the truck stops, you can really add on the minutes just by walking from your rig to the entrance of the building and back to your rig.

  - Be sure to wear a bright-colored shirt if you plan to walk around the truck stop so other drivers can easily see you.
  - Look for walking trails next to the truck stops. Just being out with nature can be energizing and a great stress reducer.

- If weather does not permit or you feel unsafe, march 10 minutes in place. Do this while watching TV or listening to music so it will be less boring. Download a fun exercise app on your phone, or access online exercise programs.

- If your balance is good, stash a small trampoline in your rig and march or jog on it for 10 minutes. This activity can be less jarring on your knees.

- If you are able to mount your bike on a rack on your rig, bike 10 minutes to add more variety to your physical activity.

Days Off

Take advantage of your days off to spend more time getting physically active by doing the following:

- Spend at least 30 minutes daily in an activity that you really enjoy such as biking, hiking, kayaking, boxing, or dancing.
- Exercise with family or friends; you will keep each other motivated.
- Park as far away as possible from the entrances to buildings in public lots.
- Do vigorous house and yard chores such as vacuuming, sweeping, raking the leaves, gardening, and pushing a lawn mower.
- Join a community Bike- or Walk-a-thon to raise money for charity while improving your fitness level.

Activity/Step Trackers and Phone Apps

If you need a motivator, track your steps and activity using technology. Keep track of the number of steps you take in your normal day.

Set a goal to try to increase your steps by 500 – 1000 steps each week. If you walk 10,000 steps in a day, you have actually walked 5 miles! Thirty-two times around an 18-wheeler is one mile, or 2,000 steps.

Other Tips

- Use truck stop gyms or fitness rooms at some chain hotels.
- Try yoga to improve your flexibility and balance. Yoga also provides stress relief and relaxation. A yoga mat is lightweight and requires minimal space.
- Remember: Give yourself a small non-food reward every time you reach a new exercise goal.

Chapter 10:

Other Healthy Lifestyle Changes

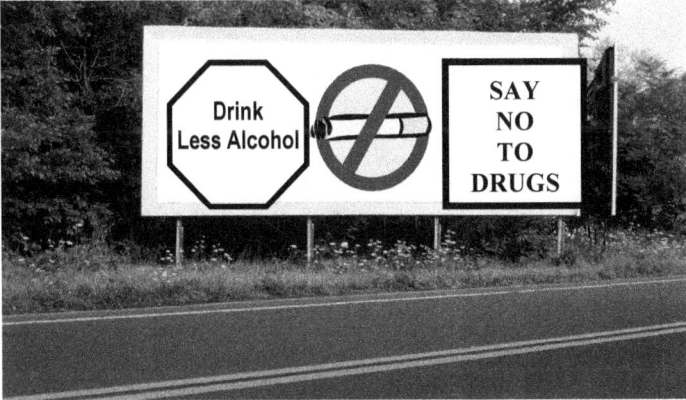

In addition to changing your diet and beginning exercise, there are other habits you can change to improve your health. Do your best to make all the changes necessary to become a healthier *you*. Read on for more information about alcohol, tobacco, drugs, and stress.

Drink Less Alcohol or Quit Drinking

According to the American Heart Association, drinking too much alcohol can raise triglycerides (blood fats), lead to high blood pressure and heart failure, and provide too many calories, which can lead to obesity and a higher risk of developing diabetes (1). In addition, binge drinking can lead to a stroke.

STOP YOUR JOB FROM KILLING YOU

If You Already Drink Alcohol

If you already drink alcohol, you may be wondering how much alcohol is safe to consume. See the following guide on alcohol use:

- The American Heart Association recommends limiting alcohol intake to one to two drinks per day for men and one drink per day for women (1).

- One *drink* is one 12-ounce beer, four ounces of wine, 1.5 ounces of 80-proof spirits, or one ounce of 100-proof spirits.

- Consult your doctor on the benefits and risks of consuming alcohol in moderation.

*If You Do **Not** Drink Alcohol*

If you don't drink alcohol, the American Heart Association cautions people **not** to start drinking since drinking excessive alcohol increases your risk for alcoholism, high blood pressure, obesity, stroke, breast cancer, suicide, and accidents (1). Also, the American Heart Association says it is not possible to predict in which people alcoholism will become a problem (1).

If You Have a Problem with Alcohol

If you have a problem with drinking, seek help now. Talk to your doctor and seek out support such as counseling or groups like Alcoholics Anonymous (AA) – look online for the local

AA phone number or visit AA.org. If you ever feel like harming yourself, call 911 and seek out medical assistance and counseling immediately.

Quit Smoking, Using Tobacco, Using Drugs

It is not new information that using tobacco and drugs is bad for your health. So, talk to your doctor and seek out help or counseling to stop your addiction. According to the American Cancer Society, there is no one right way to quit, but there are some key steps in quitting tobacco successfully, including:

1. Making the decision to quit.
2. Setting a quit date and choosing a quit plan.
3. Managing withdrawal.
4. Staying "quit" – staying tobacco-free for life (2).

You can visit Cancer.org for more information.

When You Quit, You May Want to Eat

When you quit using tobacco, drugs, or alcohol, you may want to eat more or replace your old habits with eating. Resist the urge! Overeating will only cause weight gain and a new bad habit. Eat when you are hungry, and stop when you are full. When you have a "craving" for your old habit, do something else. The American Cancer Society provides a long list of ways to combat cravings at: Cancer.org (Search 'Cravings.')

Some of the American Cancer Society's Tips for Combating Cravings

- If you miss the feeling of having something in your mouth, try toothpicks, cinnamon sticks, sugarless gum, celery, or carrots instead of constantly eating or choosing snack foods.
- Instead of drinking beverages you associate with your old habit, drink water or unsweetened, decaffeinated teas.
- Eat several small meals during the day instead of one or two large ones to keep your blood sugar levels constant, to keep your energy balanced, and to help prevent the urge to smoke. Keep hydrated, too.
- Avoid sugary or spicy foods that may trigger a desire for cigarettes.
- Stay active with sports, activities, hobbies, or by spending time with others who support your quit efforts.
- Try to choose only smoke-free restaurants and bars.
- Reward yourself for doing your best: Plan to do something fun (go fishing, shopping, or bowling) and give yourself non-food rewards (buy something special for yourself with all the money you saved **not** buying cigarettes or tobacco products) (3).

Put the Brakes on Stress

People react to stress in many different ways. While some people lose their appetite when stressed, others may overeat or overindulge on snack foods. When overeating or eating less healthy foods, other problems can arise like gaining weight or not getting the right nutrients.

The Best Diet for Stress

The best diet for stress is the one we told you about in chapter 2. Get plenty of whole grains, fruits, vegetables, lean meats, poultry, and fish, and moderate amounts of healthy fats from foods like olive oil and nuts. Drink plenty of water, and exercise to blow off some steam. Here are some other tips for staying healthy when stressed:

- Do not skip meals: Eat healthy, balanced meals throughout the day.
- Eat breakfast.
- Plan for snacks so you make healthy choices and so you don't get too hungry.
- For snacks, think plants: cucumber, apple, or orange slices.
- Take one serving of a snack, put this amount on a plate or in a baggie, and put the rest away. This will help you avoid overeating or emotional eating.
- Keep the healthy choices out on the counter or in the front of the fridge, and save the less healthy foods for once in a while.
- Drink lots of water and caffeine-free, unsweetened drinks.
- Sit down to eat, turn off the TV, and enjoy each bite.
- Eat with family and friends.

- Exercise to release stress – go for a walk, lift weights, or try some yoga.
- Enjoy the company of friends and family for a movie, a phone conversation, or another enjoyable activity. Stay connected even when you are on the road.
- Get enough sleep. Take 20-minute power naps when needed to improve mood, alertness, and performance (4).
- Organize your schedule, your home, and your workspace.
- Finally, plan ahead and be prepared.
  - For example, plan ahead by bringing healthy snacks to work.
  - Or, plan ahead by making a weekly menu of foods that you will prepare, which will also help you make a grocery list with the items you will need for the week.

References

1. American Heart Association. Alcohol and heart health. Available at: Heart.org. Accessed May 13, 2019.
2. American Cancer Society. Deciding to quit smoking and making a plan. Available at: Cancer.org. Accessed May 13, 2019.
3. American Cancer Society. Quitting smoking: Help for cravings and tough situations. Available at: Cancer.org. Accessed May 13, 2019.
4. National Sleep Foundation. Napping. Sleepfoundation.org. Accessed May 13, 2019.

Our Final Thoughts

We, the authors, hope you have found this book both useful and motivational. We encourage you to use the information that best meets your needs to ultimately improve your health and your life. Good luck and best wishes to you as you begin your journey down the road to a more healthful life.

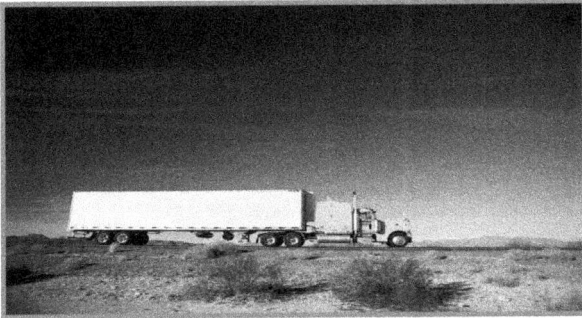

Appendix A:

12 Fast Facts for Drivers in the Fast Lane

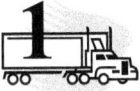

It is hard to stay healthy when you are a truck driver. But you can do it if you want to! Truckers are important to America so learn how to take care your health!

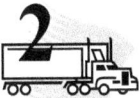

Go to ChooseMyPlate.gov for personalized diet information. Aim for three MyPlate meals a day using the following guidelines:

- Fruit: 2 cups a day
- Vegetables: 3 cups a day
- Grains: 6 ounces a day
- Milk: 3 cups a day
- Meat and meat substitutes: 6 ounces a day
- Fats: 6 servings a day

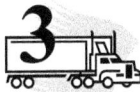

Watch your portions. Use your fist to represent the size of a serving of fruits, vegetables, grains, or milk. The palm of your hand should be your meat portion, and your thumb or small fingertip equals your fat servings.

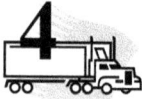

4 Choose baked, grilled, or broiled items. Avoid any fried foods. Start your meal with a vegetable salad with dressing on the side or a steaming hot broth-based soup such as vegetable soup. Eat seconds of vegetables, but watch the butter and cream sauces.

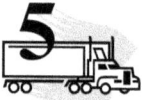

5 Stock your cab with healthier foods that are packed with energy. Consider adding a small refrigerator to your rig to give you more healthy food options.

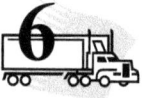

6 To lose weight, choose three MyPlate meals a day on a smaller plate. Eat breakfast every day, and try to eat meals every four to five hours.

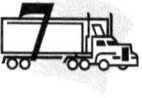

7 If you are counting calories, follow these simple guidelines:

- Entrees: less than 500 calories
- Side dishes including desserts: less than 200 calories
- Snacks: less than 200 calories
- Beverages: less than 100 calories.
- Remember, water is calorie-free.

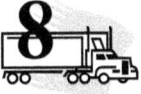

8 Get your cholesterol levels and blood pressure checked to keep your heart healthy.

- Reduce the fat in your diet (particularly saturated and trans fats).
- Eat less salt and high sodium foods and more potassium-rich foods such as fresh fruits and vegetables.
- Choose foods with less than 140 mg of sodium per serving and less than 500 mg per meal.

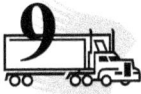

9 Get your blood sugars checked. If you have pre-diabetes or diabetes, lose weight through a healthy diet and exercise. Limit sweets and sugar-containing beverages. Choose foods that have less than 25 grams of total carbohydrate per serving.

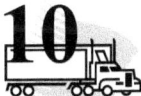

10 Stay energized the healthy way. Limit excessive caffeine and so-called "energy" pills and potions. Eat regular meals and nutritious snacks, drink plenty of water, improve sleep habits, and stay physically active.

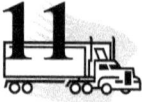

11 Cut down on screen time and increase physical activity using the "10-4" Rule. Use your smart phone or wear an activity/step tracker, and aim for 10,000 steps a day.

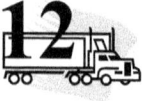

12 Learn healthier ways to manage stress. Avoid tobacco and limit the use of alcohol.

Appendix B:

Recommended Websites

General Health and Nutrition Information

- truckersnews.com -- Online newsletter for truckers; access 'health' tab

- choosemyplate.gov -- USDA individualized food guidance system; includes food and nutrition, meal planning, recipes and exercise information

- nutrition.gov -- USDA information on food and human nutrition for consumers

- eatright.org -- Food and nutrition information by the Academy of Nutrition and Dietetics

Meal Planning

- mealtime.org -- Easy, free, healthy recipes and menu planning information

Eating Out

- healthydiningfinder.com -- Resource for finding healthier restaurant choices nationwide

Weight Management

- fitday.com -- Free diet and weight loss journal

- caloriecontrol.org -- Includes a calorie calculator and a Get Moving! Calculator under Healthy Weight Tool Kit

- Mobile phone apps: Lose It! and MyFitnessPal

- Recovery Record app -- Non-calorie-based meal recording app

Fad Diets

- everydayhealth.com -- Detailed information on different fad diets including the pros and cons

Calorie Information

- calorieking.com -- Calorie and nutrient information on individual foods, including name brand and fast foods

Heart Health

- heart.org -- American Heart Association consumer information on heart-healthy eating and more

Diabetes

- diabetes.org -- Comprehensive diabetes information by the American Diabetes Association

- diabetescontrolforlife.com -- Self-management diabetes information and healthy recipes

Exercise Information

- silversneakers.com -- Search for in-person classes or on-line videos geared toward older adults

- health.gov -- Physical Activity Guidelines for Americans

- mapmyrun.com -- Map a walking or running route in any neighborhood

- go4life.nia.nih.gov-- Exercises for endurance, strength, balance and flexibility

- peertrainer.com -- Free membership to join online groups to help motivate you to meet your fitness goals

Dietary Supplements

- nccam.nih.gov/health/herbsataglance.htm -- National Center for Complementary and Alternative Medicine; health information on herbs and other dietary supplements

- ods.od.nih.gov -- National Institutes of Health vitamin, mineral and other dietary supplements fact sheets

- consumerlab.com -- Product testing, warnings, and recalls on variety of dietary supplements

Mental Health

- psychcentral.com/resources -- Mental Health and Psychology Resources Online; information on addiction and substance abuse

Appendix C:
Just for Men/Just for Women
For Men Only

Sexual problems can become more prevalent in men and women as they age. The most common problem reported by men is erectile dysfunction (ED), difficulty maintaining an erection sufficient for sex. ED is less common in men <u>without</u> chronic medical problems who engage in healthy behaviors, such as regular exercise. Conditions that put men at higher risk for ED include obesity, diabetes, chronic kidney disease, high blood pressure, heart disease, smoking, alcohol and opioid abuse and the use of some medications. While you cannot stop ED related to aging, you can take action to improve your eating and exercise habits that can help decrease your risk for sexual problems. The following are recommended guidelines for ED:

- **Manage your weight** by making healthful food choices, practicing mindful eating, decreasing portions, eating regular meals, and exercising. This can help decrease your risk for heart disease and diabetes.
- **Choose a healthier diet** with less fat, especially less saturated fat and trans fat, and less sugar and sodium. Increase fresh fruits, vegetables, whole grains, nuts and seeds in your diet.
- **You may have a poor body image** due to excess weight that keeps you from enjoying sex. Tips for safe ways to lose weight can be found in chapter 5.

- **Love yourself** as you are and work toward better nutrition for health.

- **Exercise daily** to include weight-bearing activity such as walking. Improve muscle strength and balance by lifting weights two to three times a week. Exercise to feel better and stronger in your body.

- **Avoid nicotine and limit alcohol** as these can disrupt sexual function.

- **Stress and fatigue** can sometimes cause sexual problems. Learn to reduce stress through getting support from family and friends or in counseling, exercising, trying relaxation techniques, and improving your sleep patterns. (Note: Tips for dealing with stress, including eating and exercise hints, can be found in chapter 10.)

- **While some companies promote herbal supplements** for ED, these products are unproven, unregulated, and can be expensive. These include: yohimbe, DHEA, ginkgo, ginseng, L-arginine, and even, 'herbal Viagra.' Some of them have harmful side effects such as nausea, diarrhea, increased blood pressure, and thinning of blood, which can increase the risk of bleeding. If you decide to use over-the-counter herbal remedies, check with your doctor or a registered dietitian nutritionist first.

- **If sexual problems persist**, seek guidance from a sympathetic doctor or counselor who can determine if there is a physical or psychological cause, such as anxiety or depression.

Quick ED Guidelines for Men

- Choose a healthier diet.
- Attain a healthier weight.
- Exercise daily.
- Avoid nicotine and limit alcohol.
- Reduce stress.
- Get enough rest.
- Be cautious with herbal treatments.
- Seek guidance from your doctor.

Recommended websites:

- niddk.nih.gov (Search 'Impotence.')
- familydoctor.org (Search 'Erectile Dysfunction.')
- menstuff.org (Search for 'Impotency.')
- EDCure.org

References

Mayo Clinic. Dietary supplements for erectile dysfunction: A natural treatment for ED? Available at: http://www.mayoclinic.org. Accessed December 9, 2018.

Leff, J. Can lifestyle changes improve erectile dysfunction? *Today's Dietitian*, April 2015.

Cunningham, GR, Rosen RC. Overview of male sexual dysfunction. Available at: http://uptodate.com. Accessed January 13, 2019.

For Women Only

As women age, fluctuating hormone levels occurring before, during, and after menopause may lead to physical changes in the body. As a result, women may experience annoying symptoms and develop certain conditions as they grow older. While the aging process cannot be stopped, women can take action to improve eating and exercise habits that may decrease these symptoms and reduce the risk for diseases, such as diabetes and heart disease. The following are recommended health guidelines for women.

Menopause

- **Manage your weight** by making healthful food choices, decreasing portion sizes, eating regular meals, and exercising. This can help decrease your risk for heart disease and diabetes. Losing excess weight can also improve tolerance to hot flashes.
- **Choose a healthier diet** with less fat, especially less saturated fat and trans fat, and less sugar and sodium. Increase fresh fruits, vegetables, and whole grains.
- **Aim for 1,000 milligrams (mg) of calcium daily** by eating 3 servings of dairy products such as milk, yogurt, and cheese, preferably low-fat. If you cannot achieve this, take two 500 mg calcium supplements in divided doses daily.

- **Get adequate vitamin D** through moderate sun exposure, from food sources, and from supplementation if recommended by your doctor. Include vitamin D-fortified milk, other vitamin D-fortified foods (check the food label), eggs, and fatty fish such as tuna or salmon in your diet regularly. If you decide to take a supplement, take 600 to 1000 IU of vitamin D-3 daily.

- **Phytoestrogens**, found in plant-based foods, may help relieve menopausal symptoms, such as hot flashes. These include soy products such as soybeans (edamame), soy yogurt, soymilk, and tofu, chickpeas, lentils, flaxseed, whole grains, and beans.

- **Current studies do not support the use of red clover, black cohosh, or evening primrose oil** to treat hot flashes. If you decide to take dietary or herbal supplements, discuss this with your doctor or a registered dietitian nutritionist. For serious problems with hot flashes, seek guidance from a doctor trained in women's health.

- **Limit caffeine and alcohol,** which may trigger hot flashes.

- **Exercise daily** to include weight-bearing activity such as walking. Improve muscle strength and balance by lifting weights two to three times a week. Try yoga to help with sleep and mood problems and to reduce stress.

Two recommended websites:

- menopause.org
- womenshealth.gov (Search 'Menopause.')

Sexual Dysfunction

- **You may experience sexual dysfunction** such as lack of sexual desire, impaired arousal, inability to achieve orgasm, or pain during intercourse at any time in your life. Causes of sexual dysfunction can include hormonal changes, hypertension, smoking, alcohol and opioid abuse, depression, anxiety and use of some medications. If problems persist, seek guidance from a sympathetic doctor who can determine if there is a physical or psychological cause.

- **Stress and fatigue** can sometimes cause sexual problems. Learn to reduce stress through getting support from family and friends, exercise, or trying yoga and other relaxation techniques. (Note: Tips for dealing with stress, including eating and exercise hints, can be found in chapter 10.)

- **You may have a poor body image** due to excess weight that keeps you from enjoying sex. Some women note improvements in their sex life after weight loss and beginning regular exercise.

- **Love yourself** as you are and work toward better nutrition for health.

- **Exercise daily** to include weight-bearing activity such as walking. Improve muscle strength and balance by lifting weights two to three times a week. Exercise to feel better and stronger in your body.

- **While some companies promote herbal supplements and massage oils** to enhance sexual desire, these products are unproven, unregulated and can be expensive. If you decide to use over-the-counter herbal remedies, check with your doctor or a registered dietitian nutritionist first.

Two recommended websites:

- healthywomen.org
- ashasexualhealth.org -American Sexual Health Association

Quick Menopause Guidelines:	*Quick Sexual Dysfunction Guidelines for Women:*
- Manage your weight. - Choose a healthier diet. - Aim for 1,000 mg calcium daily. - Get enough vitamin D. - Introduce soy foods like soy milk and edamame into your diet. - Be cautious with herbal supplements. - Limit caffeine and alcohol. - Exercise daily.	- Talk to your doctor to determine if there is a physical or psychological cause. - Reduce stress. - Get enough rest. - Attain a healthy weight. - Exercise. - Be cautious with herbal supplements.

References

Cleveland Clinic. Menopause topics under Health Library. Available at: my.clevelandclinic.org. Accessed January 15, 2019.

Collins SC. Boomer health: weight gain and menopause. *Today's Dietitian.* February 2015.

Shifren JL. Sexual dysfunction in women: Management. Available at www.uptodate.com. Accessed January 15, 2019.

Thalheimer JC. Women's health: are menopause supplements effective? *Today's Dietitian.* March 2016.

Appendix D:

Nutrition Therapy to Prevent Kidney Stones

Some conditions we discussed in this book can make you prone to forming kidney stones. These include diabetes, obesity, and high blood pressure. Being prone to kidney stones can also be an inherited condition. If you have kidney stones, seek guidance from a doctor who specializes in treating kidney stones. The following nutrition therapy can help prevent kidney stones:

- Drink more fluids – <u>at least</u> 64 ounces a day. Water is the best fluid. To meet this goal, drink at least 10 ounces of fluid at each meal, between meals, and at bedtime.

- Avoid large quantities of any of the following fluids: grapefruit juice, sports drinks, teas, sodas and other beverages containing "phosphoric acid" such as colas, Dr. Pepper®, and some root beers. Also avoid foods with added phosphorus by looking at the ingredient list on the label.

- Food sources of citric acid can help prevent kidney stones. Include good sources of citric acid in your diet regularly such as lemonade, lemon water, lemons, and limes.

- Limit sodium to less than 2,000 milligrams (mg) a day. You can achieve this goal by avoiding the use of salt and limiting these foods: processed luncheon meats and cheese, hot dogs, bacon, sausage, canned soups and other packaged convenience foods, salted snacks, canned vegetable juices, sports drinks, and fast food. Choose foods that have less than 140 mg of sodium per serving.

- Include two to three servings of good sources of calcium in your diet every day. A serving is: 8 ounces milk, 8 ounces yogurt, 1 ½ ounce cheese (preferably aged cheese such as cheddar), 8 ounces calcium-fortified orange juice.

- Limit high oxalate foods: spinach, beets, rhubarb, French fries, potato chips, instant tea and chocolate.

- Avoid large portions of meat, poultry, and fish. Keep portions of meat to no more than the size of the palm of your hand, and limit to twice a day. Also avoid high protein diets.

- Talk to your doctor before taking dietary supplements such as vitamin C, vitamin D, calcium supplements, or over-the-counter antacids containing calcium.

Reference

Mahan LK. Krause's Food & the Nutrition Care Process, 14th ed., 2017.

Appendix E:

Trucker's Grocery List (may be copied for use)

Fruits - Eat at least 2 cups every day.		Grains - Eat at least 6 ounces every day. Choose those that have a "whole" grain listed as the first ingredient, such as "whole wheat."	
□ Apples	□ Papaya	□ Whole grain cereal	□ Barley
□ Apricots	□ Pineapple	□ Oatmeal	□ Lentils
□ Bananas	□ Plums	□ Bread, whole wheat	□ Beans (kidney, pinto,
□ Blueberries	□ Strawberries	□ Flour tortilla, high fiber	chick peas, black
□ Cantaloupe	□ Watermelon	□ Pita, whole grain	beans, and more.)
□ Cherries	□ Frozen fruit	□ English muffin, grain	□ Pretzels
□ Grapes	without added sugar	□ Small bagel, wheat	□ Light popcorn
□ Kiwis	□ Canned or jarred	□ Small fruit muffin	□ Quinoa
□ Mango	fruit without added	□ Rice, brown	□ _____
□ Nectarine	sugar	□ Pasta, wheat	□ _____
□ Oranges	□ Dried fruit	□ Crackers, whole grain	□ _____
□ Peaches	□ _____	**Protein** - Eat 6 ounces every day.	
□ Pears	□ _____	□ Skinless chicken	□ Cheese
Vegetables - Eat at least 3 cups every day.		□ Skinless turkey	□ Peanut butter
		□ Fish/shellfish	□ Nut butters
□ Asparagus	□ Mushrooms	□ Venison	□ Hummus
□ Avocados	□ Onions	□ Lean beef/pork	□ Edamame
□ Broccoli	□ Peas	□ Eggs	□ Low sodium lunch
□ Brussels	□ Potatoes	□ Tofu	meats
sprouts	□ Spinach		□ _____
□ Cabbage	□ Squash	**Fats** - Limit to a few servings a day.	
□ Carrots	□ Sweet potatoes	□ Tub margarine	□ Walnuts
□ Cauliflower	or yams	□ Vegetable oil (such as	□ Almonds
□ Celery	□ Tomatoes	olive or canola oils)	□ Sunflower seeds
□ Corn	□ Zucchini	□ Mayonnaise	□ Flaxseeds
□ Eggplant	□ Frozen	□ Salad dressing	□ Olives
□ Green beans	vegetables	□ Sour cream	□ _____
□ Green or red	□ 'No salt added'	□ Neufchatel cream	□ _____
peppers	canned vegetables	cheese	□ _____
□ Lettuce (dark	□ Tomato or	□ Peanuts	
green, leafy)	vegetable juices	**Snacks and Beverages** - Limit snacks to only a few servings daily.	
□ Lima beans	□ _____		
Dairy - Include 3 servings every day.			
□ Low-fat milk	□ Cheese	□ Baked potato chips	□ Water
□ Soy or dairy-	□ Low-fat ice	□ Animal crackers	□ Flavored water (diet)
free milks	cream	□ Single serve snack	□ Diet tea
□ Yogurt	□ String cheese	packs	□ Diet soda
□ GoGurt®	□ Cottage cheese	□ Beef jerky	□ _____
□ Light pudding			

Index

About the Authors

SHARON MADALIS, MS, RDN, LDN, CDE

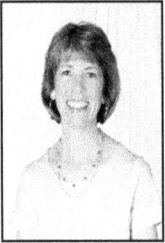

Sharon Madalis is a Registered Dietitian Nutritionist who counsels clients in a variety of outpatient clinics for Geisinger in central Pennsylvania. From her experiences as a dietitian, she became inspired to create a series of nutrition books focused on promoting healthier lifestyles for people in occupations with difficult and stressful work environments. Sharon has an undergraduate degree in Medical Dietetics from Penn State University and a Master's degree in Instructional Technology from Bloomsburg University. She is a Certified Diabetes Educator and holds a Certificate of Training in Adult Weight Management through the Academy of Nutrition and Dietetics/Commission on Dietetic Registration. Sharon is not only excited to start the series with this book but also to be collaborating on the book with one of her former interns, April Rudat.

APRIL RUDAT, MS Ed, RDN, LDN

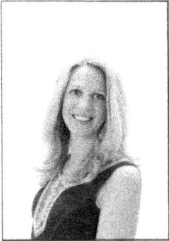

April Rudat is a Registered Dietitian Nutritionist in private practice and works as a writer, speaker, and nutrition counselor for adults, children, and families who want to attain a healthier lifestyle (DietitianApril.com). She is also a "non-diet" dietitian and is a passionate advocate for the prevention and treatment of eating disorders. April is also the author of the book, "Oh Yes You Can Breastfeed Twins!" which published in 2007 and has sold over 2,000 copies. She also works as part-time adjunct faculty at Marywood University in Scranton, PA. April has a Master's degree in Counseling from Old Dominion University in Norfolk, VA, and she received her undergraduate degree from Indiana University of Pennsylvania in Indiana, PA. She completed her dietetic internship experience at Geisinger Medical Center in Danville, PA, under the supervision of Sharon Madalis. She also holds a Certificate of Training in Adult Weight Management through the Academy of Nutrition and Dietetics/Commission on Dietetic Registration.

www.ingramcontent.com/pod-product-compliance
Lightning Source LLC
Chambersburg PA
CBHW071133280326
41935CB00010B/1213